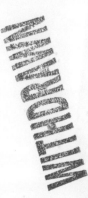

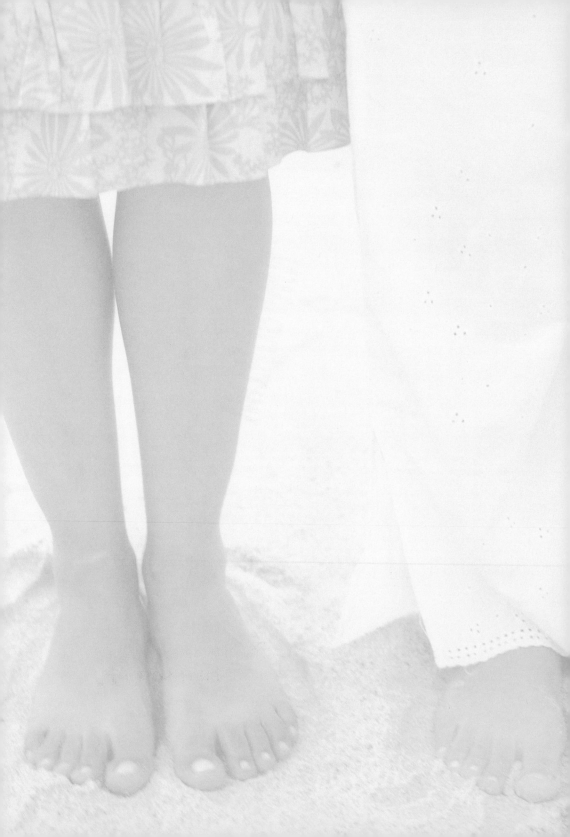

perfect feet

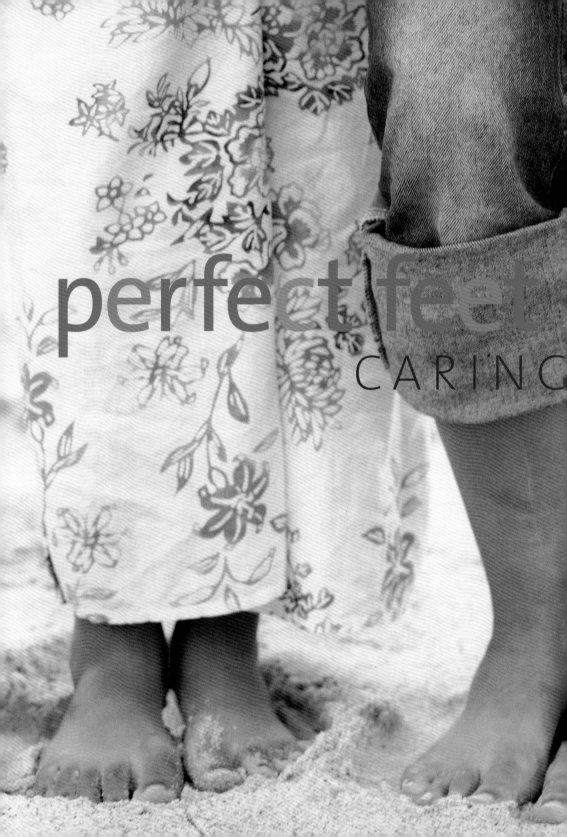

ND PAMPERING

DR. STUART MOGUL
written with Jacqueline deMontravel

PHOTOGRAPHS BY ERICKA MCCONNELL

stewart, tabori & chang
NEW YORK

Text copyright © 2002 Dr. Stuart Mogul
and Jacqueline deMontravel

Photographs copyright © 2002 Ericka McConnell
STYLIST • Loren Simons
LOCATIONS • Jody and Giulio Martini's home in
Sagaponick, New York and Patrick Orban's Soho
loft in New York City
ACCESSORIES • The following items are available from
the sources listed. Courtesy of Sigerson Morrison,
New York: shoes on pages 79 and 85; Courtesy of
Niketown.com: running shoes on page 34.

"Ten Points of Proper Shoe Fit" on page 81,
copyright © 1992, 1999, National Shoe Retailers
Association, Columbia, MD. Reprinted with permission.
For shoe fit assistance, please contact a retailer via Shoe
Search at www.nsra.org, or a certified pedorthist via
www.pedorthics.org.

EDITORS • Sandy Gilbert and Elaine Schiebel
PRODUCTION • Alexis Mentor
DESIGNER • Alexandra Maldonado

Published by
STEWART, TABORI & CHANG
A Company of La Martinière Groupe
115 West 18th Street
New York, NY 10011

Export Sales to all countries except
Canada, France, and French-speaking Switzerland:
Thames and Hudson Ltd.
181A High Holborn
London WC1V 7QX
England

Canadian Distribution:
Canadian Manda Group
One Atlantic Avenue, Suite 105
Toronto, Ontario M6K 3E7
Canada

Library of Congress Cataloging-in-Publication Data
Mogul, Stuart.
    Perfect feet : caring and pampering / by Stuart
Mogul and Jacqueline deMontravel.
        p. cm.
    ISBN 1-58479-278-7
1. Foot—Care and hygiene. I. deMontravel,
Jacqueline. II. Title.

RD563 .M684 2003
617.5'85—dc21
                2002036452

The text of this book was composed in Avenir.
Printed in Hong Kong
10 9 8 7 6 5 4 3 2 1
First Printing

ACKNOWLEDGMENTS

I would like to thank the many
patients who entrusted the care
of their feet to me. Allowing me
to use my skills and knowledge
as a surgeon to relieve their
suffering has been as much an
honor and privilege today as it
was eighteen years ago when I
started my practice.

I would also like to thank my
mother and father who encour-
aged me to fulfill my dreams of
becoming a doctor. Thank you to
my loving wife Valerie and our
three children, who gave me the
time and space to write.

My special thanks to Jacqueline
deMontravel, Sandy Gilbert,
Meryl Jacobs, Elaine Schiebel,
Lance Warrick, Jody and Giulio
Martini, Dr. Sherman Nagler,
Alexandra Maldonado, and Ericka
McConnell who all helped immea-
surably in creating this book.

—Stuart Mogul

Publishers Note: The remedies contained within this book are in no way intended as a substitute for medical counseling. Please do not attempt self-treatment for foot ailments without first consulting a medical professional or qualified practitioner.

Thanks to Stuart, Sandy, Elaine, and Meryl for keeping to foot patrol. Special thanks to Dr. Debra Jaliman, Dr. Laurie Polis, Marcia Kilgore of Bliss Spa, Beth Mann, and Regine Berthelot of Frédéric Fekkai who helped me stay on the right path. To Deborah Geltman, Victoria van Vlaanderen, Joanne Napolitano, and Greg and Constance Dalvito who stood by me. And to my Mother who gave me my royal toes—albeit webbed ones.

–Jacqueline deMontravel

contents

FIVE STEPS TO THE PERFECT FEET

INTRODUCTION

Around two million years ago, a profound cascade of events unfolded when the first hominids began to use hands solely for grasping instead of walking. Standing erect, as opposed to bearing weight on all four limbs, gave our aboriginal ancestors a distinct advantage over their four-legged contemporaries. For example, vision was no longer directed toward the ground, so they could effortlessly scan more than 180 degrees in each direction.

In fact, the transformation from quadrupeds to bipeds is a very large and important piece of an evolutionary puzzle that set us on a path toward the computer-using, city-building, and high-heel-wearing women we eventually became.

All of these improvements, however, came with a price. When our body weight was shifted onto two limbs instead of four, we doubled the pressure placed on the most earthbound parts of our body: our feet. Shortly after (on the evolutionary time scale), we began to ensconce our taxed feet in sandals, shoes, and boots of every size and shape imaginable, putting the axiom "form follows function" into questionable balance.

Although we walk, run, and dance with our heads held high, our feet are constant reminders of our most humble beginnings. One of my patients framed our painful relationship with our most terminal appendages fittingly when she asked, "How can we send a man to the moon and still have feet that hurt so much?"

The answer to this question is not a short or easy one. Podiatric and orthopedic surgeons have made great leaps in recent years in the biomechanical under-standing of how the foot does what it does, as well as what happens when things go to hell in a handbasket and our patients cry from "agony of de feet."

Today's foot specialists are better equipped to identify specific foot problems faster and more accurately, thanks to modern imaging techniques such as magnetic resonance imaging (MRI) and computed tomography (CT) scanning. Computerized gait analysis can provide valuable clues to pathological processes that occur as the foot is moving from step to step. Surgical techniques, biomaterials, and advanced med-ical equipment have made the outcome of foot surgery for deformities such as bunions, corns, and hammertoes more predictable and less painful than in the past. Cosmetic foot surgery, once unthinkable, is now becom-ing a new and exciting area, focusing on the aesthetics of the human foot and freeing patients not only from painful but embarrassing foot anomalies as well.

It is this science of diagnosing and treating a part of our anatomy that has undergone such a recent evolu-tionary growth spurt that drew me to become a foot surgeon in the first place. Using my hands to counter the effects of gravity and time on another person's feet is a profound and rewarding experience. I have drawn upon almost two decades of clinical experi-ence with the complexities and workings of the human foot to write this book.

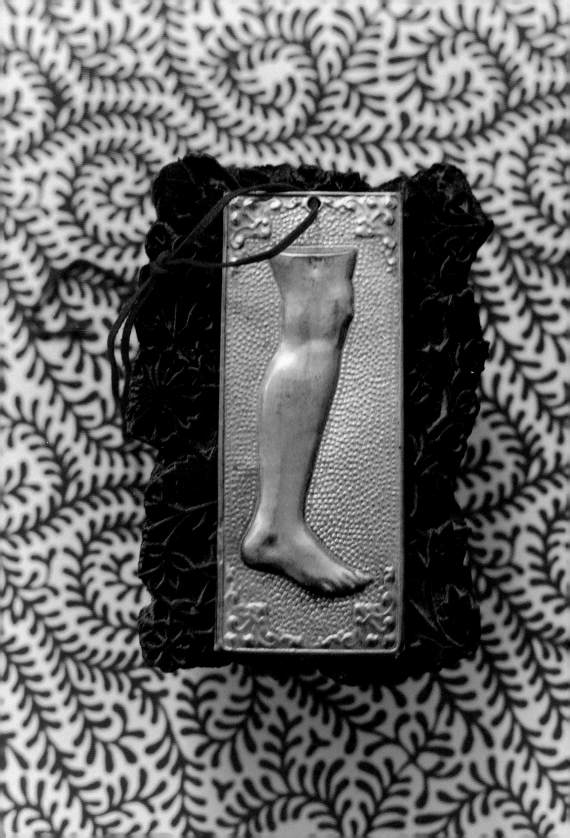

step 1
your feet

UNDERSTANDING AI

The foot, like a beautifully and ingeniously designed building, is both complex and functional. It is the most elaborate structure in the human body and is made up of 28 bones, 33 joints, 107 ligaments, 31 tendons, and miles of nerves and blood vessels. Half of all the bones in your body are in the feet.

Even the skin covering the feet is highly specialized. If you think of the skin of the body as fine silk, then the skin on the feet would be Gorertex®—four times as thick. When treated with care, this complicated network of components will never let you down, but like a building that falls into disrepair, neglect will take its toll on your feet.

THE FOOT'S FUNCTION

The foot has two main functions: to support the body's weight and to seamlessly transfer that weight onto a variety of surfaces with each step. It must be at once a loose bag of bones to adapt to varied surfaces and a sturdy platform that is capable of propelling your body weight forward. This is the yin and the yang of the foot—its two seemingly opposite natures that are both necessary in order for it to work properly. The foot's twiglike bones interlock like jigsaw puzzle pieces, which lock and unlock according to the foot's activity. This is called *pronation,* when the foot is unlocked and flexible; and *supination,* when it is locked and rigid. The foot's ability to recognize and adapt to different surfaces is what keeps us from wobbling like penguins.

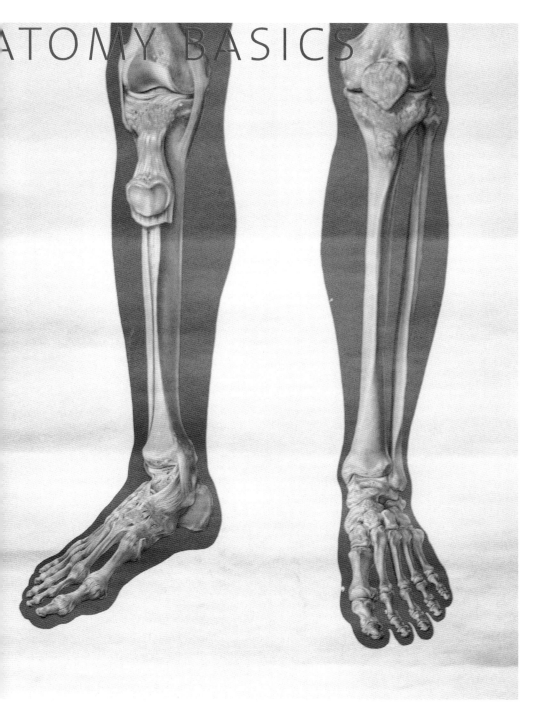

DETERMINING YOUR FOOT TYPE

FOOT STRUCTURE

The foot is composed of three sections—the forefoot (the toes), midfoot (the arch), and hindfoot (the heel).

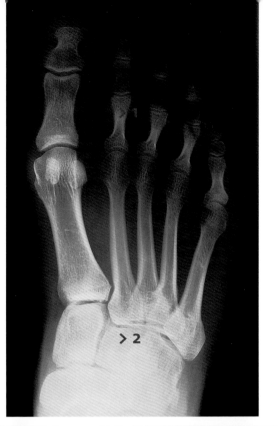

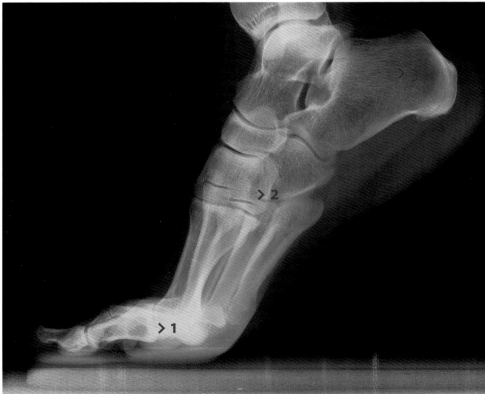

1 > THE FOREFOOT

The forefoot includes the five metatarsal bones, and the phalanges (the toes). The first metatarsal bone bears the most weight and plays the most important role in propulsion. The shortest and thickest, it also provides attachment for several tendons. The second, third, and fourth metatarsal bones are the most stable of the metatarsals. They are well protected and have only minor tendon attachments. Near the head of the first metatarsal, on the plantar surface of the foot, are two sesamoid bones (a small, oval-shaped bone that develops inside a tendon where the tendon passes over a bony prominence). They are held in place by their tendons, and are also supported by ligaments.

2 > THE MIDFOOT

The midfoot includes five of the seven tarsal bones (the navicular, the cuboid, and the three cuneiform). The distal row contains the three cuneiforms and the cuboid. The midfoot meets the forefoot at the five tarsometatarsal joints. There are multiple joints within the midfoot. The three cuneiforms articulate with the navicular bone.

3 > THE HINDFOOT

The talus and the calcaneus make up the hindfoot. The calcaneus is the largest tarsal bone, and forms the heel. The talus rests on top of it, and forms the pivotal, lower half of the ankle joint.

The two most common shapes of the human foot are the *plano-valgus,* or flat foot, and the *cavus,* or high-arched foot.

THE FLAT FOOT

The flat foot easily adapts to various ground surfaces, yet has a difficult time transferring weight from one foot to the other during a normal walking gait. The flat foot is in the pronated (flexible) phase through all phases of the walking gait cycle—from the moment the heel strikes the ground to the final push from the toes that leads to the next step. This lack of rigidity overworks muscles and tendons in the foot and leg, which become worn out in the attempt to make the foot more rigid. The demands placed on these muscles are often expressed as arch and leg fatigue after walking, running, or even standing in place for long periods of time. Beyond the symptoms of fatigue, a flat foot puts undue stress on various joints in the foot. It is not surprising that severely flat feet often undergo arthritic changes in several of the foot's joints.

HIGH-ARCHED FOOT

The high-arched foot makes contact with the ground over a smaller area than the flat foot, mainly with the ball and heel. Because of the concentration of weight on a smaller surface, people with high-arched feet often complain of soreness and calluses on the ball and heel.

Additionally, because of the position of a joint called the *subtalar*, the foot becomes more rigid. This joint, located underneath the ankle joint, functions to pronate and supinate the foot. High-arched feet have difficulty adapting to uneven surfaces as well as absorbing shock. As a result, people with high-arched feet are more susceptible to ankle sprains. Calluses are a common problem for people with high-arched feet. Knee, hip, and back pain may also occur due to poor shock absorption.

> To determine your foot type, wet the bottom of your foot and stand on an eight-by-twelve inch sheet of cardboard or, if you have access to a beach, make a clear imprint of your foot on firmly packed, moist sand. If the wet print of your foot covers the entire length of your footprint, from heel to toes, you have a flat foot. If there is an area between the ball and heel of your footprint that is completely dry from side to side, you have a high-arched foot.

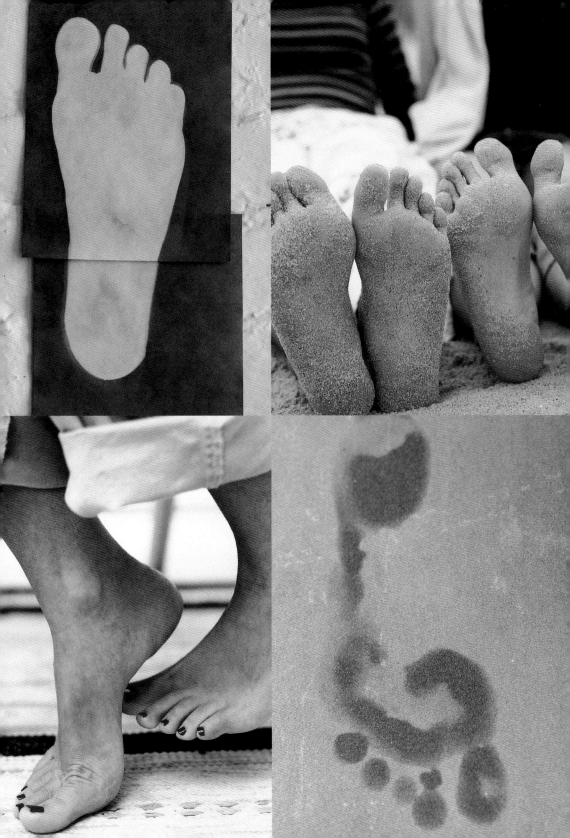

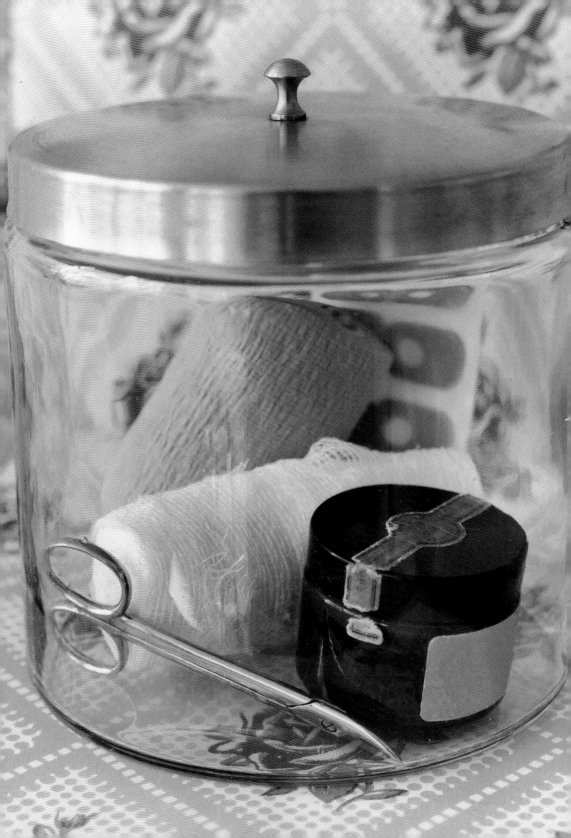

step 2
caring

CONDITIONS, TREATM

For many of us who suffer from foot problems, going barefoot in public is a feat in itself. Those cratered nubs, cartoonlike toe bulges, and reptilelike skin can be an embarrassment and a sight we wouldn't want to reveal to others. However, ignoring foot problems can not only lead to embarrassment but also serious and costly medical problems.

Whether painful to the eye or simply painful, the following are some of the most common foot problems and ways to treat and prevent them.

ATHLETE'S FOOT

Athlete's foot is a fungus infection. The fungi that cause athlete's foot are like small mushrooms that multiply in dark, damp places. Everyone is susceptible to athlete's foot, but unless the growing conditions are ideal the infection is not likely.

Athlete's foot is indicated in a variety of ways. For some, the skin between the toes (especially the last two toes), peels, cracks, and becomes scaly. For others, there is redness, scaling, and blisters on the soles and along the sides of the feet. Often these skin changes are accompanied by itching and burning. Toenail infections can also occur and are typically very stubborn to treat. These infections result in scaling, crumbling, and thickening of the nails and can also result in nail loss.

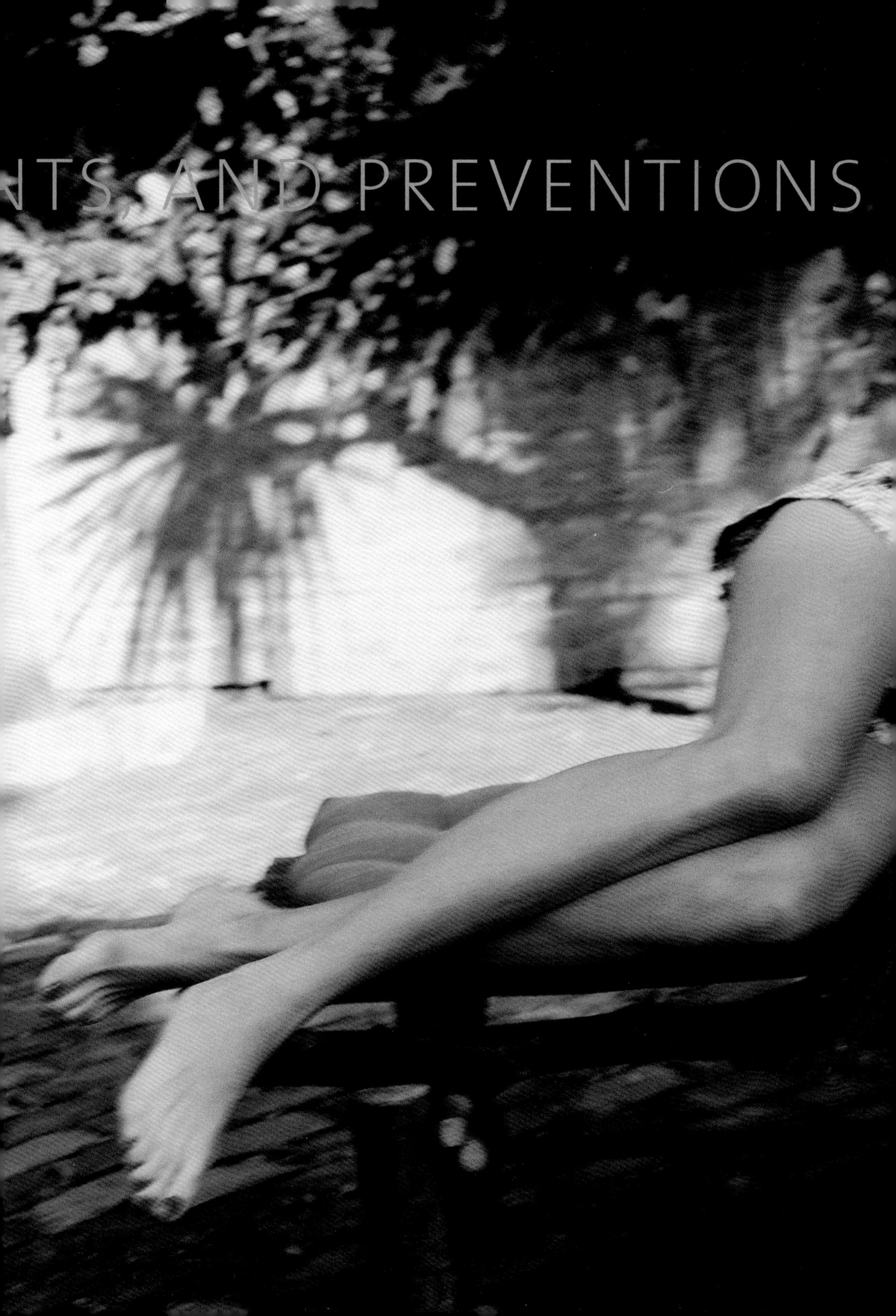
NTS, AND PREVENTIONS

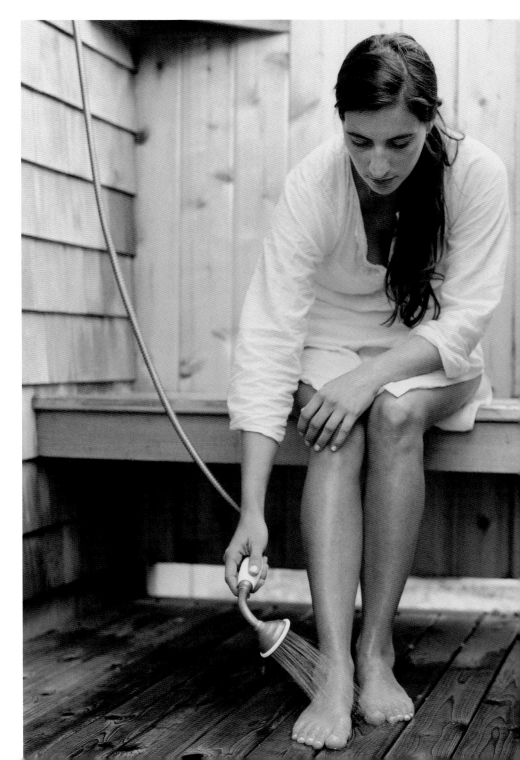

TREATMENT   As not all rashes on the feet are athlete's foot, it's prudent to have your foot specialist or dermatologist properly diagnose the condition and prescribe the correct medication. Using over-the-counter products on a rash that is not athlete's foot may make your condition worse.

Once the fungus is diagnosed, your doctor can prescribe an antifungal cream to remedy simple cases. In more severe cases, your foot specialist and dermatologist may prescribe foot soaks before applying antifungal creams (see page 61). If your athlete's foot is stubborn, antifungal pills are also available. If athlete's foot isn't treated, the skin blisters and cracks can lead to bacterial infections.

As with all medications, it's important to continue the use of your prescribed antifungal creams and to take all medication even if the condition seems to have improved or healed. While your skin may look better, the infection can remain for some time afterward and could recur.

PREVENTION

> Wash your feet daily. If you are prone to athlete's foot, wash your feet twice a day and dry them thoroughly, especially in between your toes.

> Wear shoes like flip-flops in places that fungi like to grow, such as public showers and other dark, moist places.

> Wear cotton or other natural-fiber socks and change frequently throughout the day if they become damp. Avoid shoes made with synthetic materials as well.

> Avoid tight footwear, especially in the summer. Sandals are the ideal warm weather footwear. However, it is even better to go barefoot as often as possible to allow your feet to dry out and "breathe."

BLISTERS

Blisters are fluid-filled pouches on the top of the skin. They form when the skin rubs against another surface, usually the inside of a shoe, causing friction. A tear occurs within the five upper layers of the skin, or the epidermis, and a space forms between the layers into which a clear fluid flows, filling up the space and pushing out the surface, which is still intact, causing a blister.

TREATMENT *Note: Those with diabetes or poor circulation should not self-treat and should consult a podiatrist or primary-care physician.*

The easiest way to prevent blisters is to wear shoes that fit you well. Choose shoes that fit comfortably, with about a thumb's width between your longest toe and the tip of the shoe. Narrow shoes can cause blisters on the big toe and little toe. Tight-fitting shoes can lead to blisters on the tops of the toes, while loose shoes can create blisters on the tips of the toes as they rub against the toe box of the shoe (see page 81). When trying on shoes, bring along the same socks, insoles, and orthotics that you normally wear. Since feet tend to swell during the day, shop for shoes in the afternoon or evening. Walk or jog around the store before buying shoes and then put them on again when you arrive at home to identify any areas of discomfort.

Most blisters can be self-treated, only needing medical attention if they become infected, recur frequently, form in unusual locations, or are very severe. Signs of infection include pus draining from the blister, warm and/or very red skin around the area, and red streaks leading away from the blister. Small, intact blisters that are not bothersome should be left alone since the blister's own skin, or "roof," is nature's most effective bandage. For additional protection, cover these blisters with a small adhesive bandage.

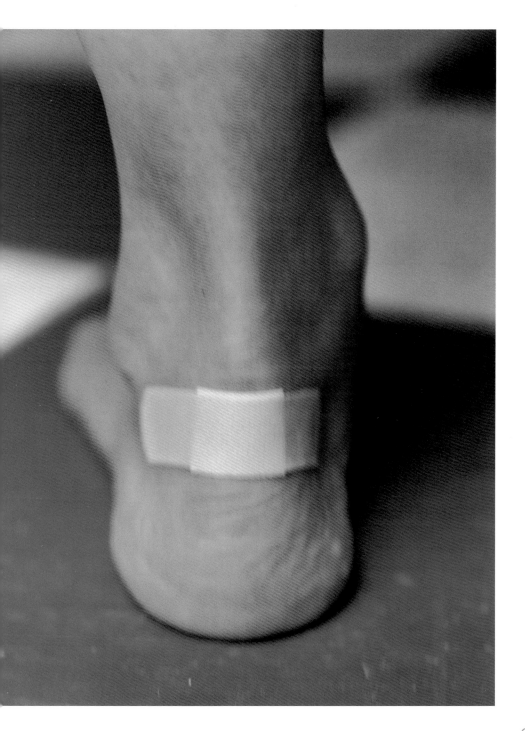

Larger or more painful blisters that are intact should be drained without removing the roof. To do this, first clean the blister with rubbing alcohol or wash with an antibiotic soap. Sterilize a straight pin over a flame until it glows red, then allow it to cool before puncturing a small hole at the edge of the blister. Drain the fluid with gentle pressure and then apply an antibiotic ointment. Cover the blister with a bandage and change the dressing daily or more frequently if it becomes wet, soiled, or loose.

Blisters with small tears should be treated the same as those that you have manually punctured. Blisters with larger tears should be "unroofed" carefully with fine scissors and the base should be cleansed thoroughly, followed by an antibiotic ointment and a bandage.

Additional padding may be necessary during exercise or sports. Ring-shaped adhesive pads made of felt can be placed on the skin around the blister, which disperses weight away from the blister. Larger blisters may require a larger sterile adhesive bandage. If you find that the bandages on your feet fall off during exercise, tape the bandage in place with either cloth or duct tape. To further decrease friction, you can also apply a thin layer of petroleum jelly to the feet underneath socks or you can apply a foot powder or foot antiperspirant spray that will keep your feet dry.

The best way to avoid discomfort is to take a break from physical activities. But if blisters do surface, prompt treatment will get you back to form quickly and help prevent infection.

> Minimize friction placed on your feet. If you know you'll be participating in an activity likely to cause blisters, such as running or wearing new shoes, you can apply a thin layer of petroleum jelly to the feet before you put on your socks.

> Keep feet dry: Foot powders and foot antiperspirant spray decrease moisture.

> Break in shoes by wearing them for 1 to 2 hours on the first day and gradually increase the amount of time you wear them.

> Wear shoes appropriate for a particular sport.

> Use cloth tape or duct tape over areas prone to blistering before you exercise or play a sport.

BOTCHED PEDICURES

Pedicures can be the source of many problems, not only of fungal infection but also of bacterial infection and hepatitis C. All are caused by the use of unsterile instruments.

TREATMENT When a nail is improperly trimmed, in many instances you have to just let it grow out. However, if you have any symptoms such as warmth, redness, or drainage from the nail, which are all signs of an infection, you must consult your foot-care specialist.

PREVENTION Do not feel inhibited to bring your own instruments to a professional manicure. It is important to feel comfortable and if you have a good relationship with your pedicurist, he/she will understand. If you do not have a good relationship, try to develop one. It is increasingly common for people to bring their own pedicure instruments with them, even at reputable salons.

BUNIONS

A bunion is a protuberance of bone and/or tissue around the big joint. A bunion at the base of the little toe or on the outside of the foot is called a "bunionette" or a "tailor's bunion."

The joint at the base of the big toe is very complex. Here the bones, tendons, and ligaments work together to distribute the body's weight. Should this joint become abnormally stressed over an extended period of time, a bunion may result. Bunions at the base of the big toe usually begin when the big toe starts moving toward the smaller toes, usually as a result of faulty biomechanics or pointy or poor-fitting shoes. Any crowding of the toes puts pressure on the joint, pushing it outward. The movement of the joint in this outward direction starts the formation of a bunion.

People with flat feet or low arches are more susceptible to bunions and should be especially wary of wearing high-heeled or improperly fitting shoes. Bunions are also associated with various forms of arthritis. Arthritis can cause the joint's protective covering of cartilage to deteriorate, leaving the joint damaged and with a decreased range of motion. For this reason, older people are more vulnerable to bunions.

Pain from a bunion can range from mild to severe, making it difficult to walk in normal shoes and, more notably, heels. The skin and deeper tissues around the bunion may also become swollen or inflamed.

A bunion can affect the other toes as the big toe pushes inward toward the smaller toes. Toenails may begin to grow into the sides of the nail bed, the smaller toes can develop corns or become bent (hammertoes), or calluses may form on the bottom of the foot.

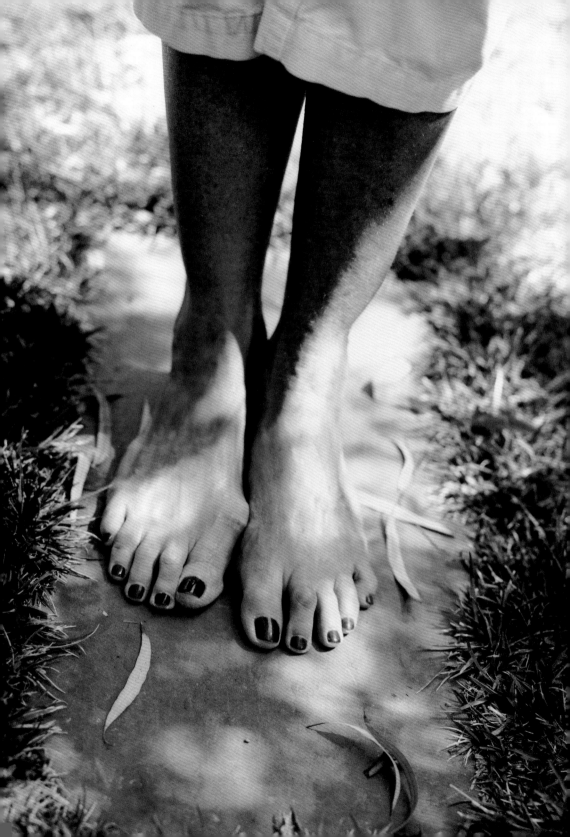

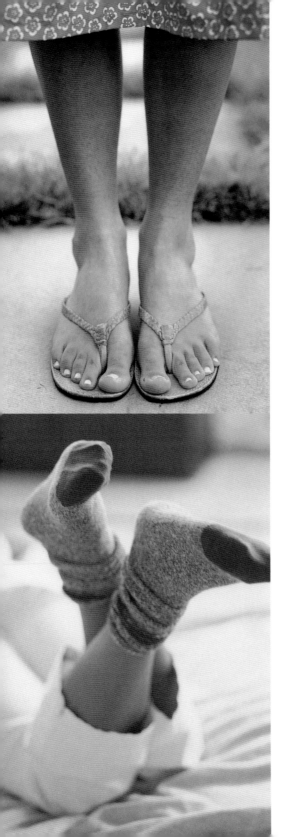

TREATMENT Treatments vary depending on the severity of pain and extent of deformity. Left untreated, bunions tend to get larger and usually more painful. An evaluation by a podiatric surgeon should be given at the first sign of pain or discomfort so that severe deformity can be prevented. The main goal of early treatment is to relieve pressure on the bunion and smaller toes and to diminish the progression of joint deformities.

Padding the bunion is an important first step, as is wearing shoes such as sandals, athletic shoes, or shoes made from soft leather that are large enough to comfortably accommodate the bunion. Stiff leather shoes may be stretched slightly for greater comfort. Tight, confining, or high-heel shoes should be avoided.

A doctor may start you on nonsteroidal anti-inflammatory drugs or cortisone injections. These prescriptions can help to ease pain and inflammation caused by joint deformities. Physical therapy, ultrasound treatment, and whirlpool baths can also provide temporary relief.

Orthotics (shoe inserts) may be useful in controlling abnormal foot movement, and may reduce symptoms for those with a painful bunion that has not yet caused a significant bony abnormality at the joint. If a systemic disease like rheumatoid arthritis or gouty arthritis is related to the bunion, appropriate medical treatment aimed at those diseases may be recommended.

When conservative treatment does not provide satisfactory relief from symptoms or when the condition interferes with physical activity, surgery is necessary. In addition to easing pain, the purpose of bunion surgery is to remove the enlargement and realign the joint to restore normal function so that the foot can carry the body's weight properly. Postoperative orthotics or support devices may be recommended to improve the foot's function.

PREVENTION

> Wear comfortable shoes as often as possible.
> See your doctor at the earliest onset of symptoms.

COLD FEET

Cold feet occur when the very small arteries in the feet (and hands) go into spasms and constrict the blood flow to the tissues. It is a common malady for women who suffer from the benign genetic condition known as Raynaud's disease. Besides feeling cold the feet may also turn a different color, from white to red to blue. Cold feet is also a symptom that occurs when other factors, such as external temperature, caffeine, and tobacco, irritate the arteries in the feet. Mild cases can be treated with warming socks, toe warmers, and precaution. Contact your doctor if any of the following occur: Your toes turn black or dusky blue, pain persists for more than two hours, red toes do not turn back to your natural color when pressure is applied to them.

CRACKED SKIN

Fissures, or deep cracks in the skin, are caused by excessively dry skin or thick calluses, usually found at the perimeter of the heel. Sandals and slingback shoes contribute to calluses and dry, cracked skin on the heel, since the heel is exposed when it spills over the back of the shoe. Fissures can be painful and may become infected unless treated.

TREATMENT Treat dry skin by rubbing the heels of the feet with a pumice stone after a shower when the skin is softer. Do not try to cut or grate rough skin yourself nor should you allow your pedicurist to smooth your skin with anything other than a pumice stone—only a podiatrist should be trusted to use a scalpel or razor blade on your foot. Finish by applying an emollient like lanolin or cream with urea; both are available over the counter at most drugstores. These creams provide a barrier and do not allow moisture to leave the skin.

PREVENTION

> Pumice dry skin regularly.

> Moisturize your feet, especially in chapped areas. Wear socks over moisturized feet to bed.

> Soak feet (see page 62).

> Avoid backless shoes.

FOOT PAIN

RUNNING

While runners swear by their highs, it doesn't often include the feet. The feet carry the weight of the entire body, and as a result active feet are more prone to problems.

It is essential for runners to wear the proper shoes (see page 86). Runners should keep their nails trimmed and inspect their feet on a regular basis. Bruises are common and typically not a problem. However, if they are persistent and frequently recur, seek medical attention.

Stretching before and after exercise can often thwart problems. If pain does occur, reduce your exercise regimen and end with a warm bath or shower and a foot massage to soothe tired muscles.

BEING OVERWEIGHT

Most people who are overweight also suffer from foot pain. Maintaining your proper weight is essential for relief from foot pain.

HAMMERTOES

A hammertoe occurs when any of the little toes curl under themselves. This happens when ligaments and tendons have tightened, causing the toe's joints to buckle, the toe to curl, and the middle part of the toe to propel upward. Shoes then rub on the prominent portion of the toe, leading to bursitis (inflammation of the joints) and eventually corns and calluses.

During its early stages, a hammertoe remains flexible, allowing it to straighten when pressure is applied to the buckled area. As time passes, however, the toe can become permanently buckled or rigid, requiring surgery for correction. Painful calluses on the bottom of the foot may accompany rigid hammertoes due to pressure generated on the joint.

TREATMENT It's important to wear shoes that comfortably accommodate the contracted toe. Your doctor may recommend a splint or pad that can hold your toes straight and felt padding that can cushion corns. If your symptoms are severe, surgery may be needed. If your joints are flexible, the tight tendon is cut and repositioned. If the joint is rigid, a piece of bone may be removed to help straighten the toe.

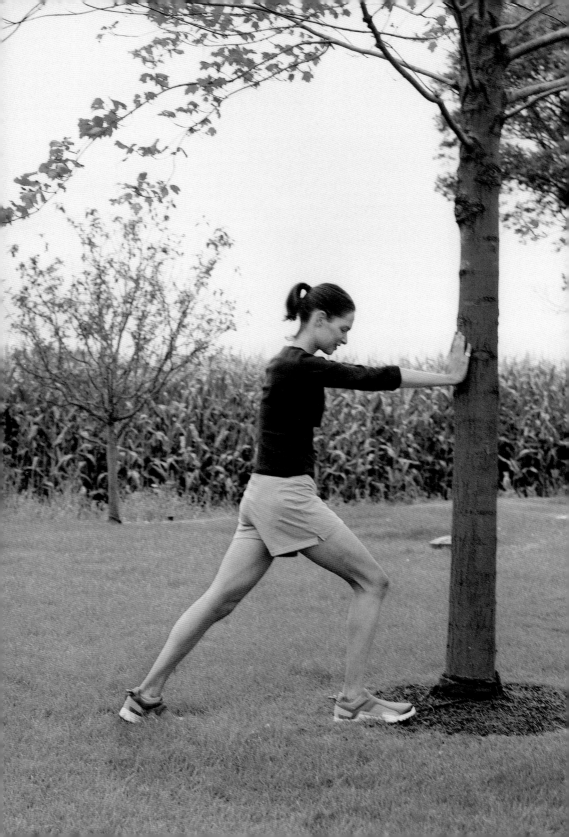

HEEL PAIN

Many people suffer from a sharp pain, aching, or stiffness on the bottom of one or both heels. This discomfort is often most intense first thing in the morning and after a period of rest or inactivity. The pain may cause people to hobble or limp for a few minutes while their feet adjust to a comfortable stride. The pain may also occur as weight is applied to heels during walking or standing.

Heel pain originates deep within the foot, directly on the heel bone or within the foot's connective tissues, called the *fascia*. Several layers of fatty tissue surround the heel bone, softening the impact of walking and running and protecting the bones and muscles of the foot. Beneath this padding the fascia extends from the heel bone all the way to the toes, and acts as an arch support in between. Pain can result when the fascia become irritated or inflamed. This inflammation may cause a heel spur to grow on the heel bone (see page 36).

TREATMENT Heel pain can be avoided, and cured, with simple stretches that are also beneficial in the treatment and prevention of many other foot problems. Since many foot injuries are a result of muscle and tendon imbalances, stretching some muscle groups while strengthening others can often prevent and reduce pain.

Stretches that involve the foot should concentrate on the Achilles tendon and calf muscles. The following stretches are most effective in treating these areas and should be done twice a day:

BASIC RUNNER'S STRETCH Bend one leg forward in a semi-lunge position and thrust the other leg straight back. Hold for one minute and switch legs.

STEP STRETCH Stand on a step, balancing on the balls of your feet with your heels hanging over the edge. Drop heels below the step and hold for one minute.

> Stretch at least twice daily.

> If you are more than your optimum weight, begin a weight-loss program to relieve pressure on the heels.

> Wear high heels as little as possible.

OTHER HEEL CONDITIONS

While injury, overuse, and poor-fitting shoes can cause pain or discomfort to the heel, a painful heel could also indicate a more serious condition. A few of these conditions are:

> Arthritis

> Collagen disorders

> Gout

> Heel-bone abnormalities

> Nerve injuries

> Psoriasis

> Tumors

HEEL SPURS

A projection or growth of bone is a spur. They can grow where the muscles of the foot attach to bone. While some heel spurs are painless, others result in chronic heel pain that requires medical treatment or surgery. (See also Bone Spurs, page 44.)

TREATMENT In most cases, heel spurs can be relieved without surgery. Simple treatments include alternating heel heights, taping and padding the foot, or modifying or temporarily eliminating sports and other vigorous activities. Orthotics also relieve the strain on the tissues and permit the heel to recover. Also, a stretching routine involving the Achilles tendon and calf muscles (see page 35) should be practiced three times a day—in the morning, before exercising, and in the evening.

If self-care measures fail to relieve the pain, a podiatric surgeon may recommend various treatments to reduce inflammation. Some of these may include:

> Nonsteroidal anti-inflammatory medications to reduce both pain and inflammation

> Extracorporeal Shock Wave (ESW)—a new treatment that uses high-energy shock waves to promote healing of the plantar fascia. ESW has been used for years to treat kidney stones.

> Cortisone injections

> Physical therapy—a podiatrist or physical therapist may treat heel pain with ultrasound, electrical stimulation, or hydrotherapy. Each of these methods may help reduce inflammation.

PREVENTION

> Modify daily routines to exclude activities that are stressful on the feet.

> Apply ice at first onset of pain.

> Alternate shoe height between low and high heels.

> Replace shoes, especially athletic footwear, regularly.

> Begin any new exercise regimen slowly. If you experience any pain, immediately end the exercise and consult a specialist.

> Stretch at least three times a day.

INGROWN AND THICKENED TOENAILS

Ingrown and thickened nails are common toenail disorders. Both have the same treatment and prevention programs. Ingrown nails occur when the nail grows into the surrounding skin; it is quite common in the big toe. Symptoms of an ingrown nail include redness, swelling, and infection. Thickened nails can develop through pressure from footwear, fungal infections, and various other conditions, including diabetes and psoriasis.

Sometimes a toe injury changes the nail's contour, which can lead to an ingrown toenail. Toe deformities (such as bunions, see page 28), and high-heel or pointy shoes also apply pressure between the nail and soft tissues, eventually forcing the nail to grow into the skin. Ingrown nails can be accompanied by other toe disorders, such as excess surrounding tissue or an outgrowth of bone beneath the nail. Painful ingrown nails may be congenital, caused by an overcurvature of the nail or an imbalance between the width of the nail plate and the nail bed.

TREATMENT Daily soaking in a salt bath may be recommended (see page 56), and if the toe is inflamed or infected, a topical antibiotic should be applied for three to seven days. If the infection is severe, an oral antibiotic may be prescribed.

In severe cases, surgery is often necessary to ease the pain and remove the offending nail. However, only a portion of the nail may be removed. If the entire nail is badly affected or there is a severe nail deformity, the nail plate and *matrix* (the cells that grow the nail) may be entirely removed.

PREVENTION

> Cut your nails straight across. Do not cut the nail too short; leave a bit of the white tip, and trim them often so they do not get too long.

> Wear well-fitting shoes with low to moderate heels.

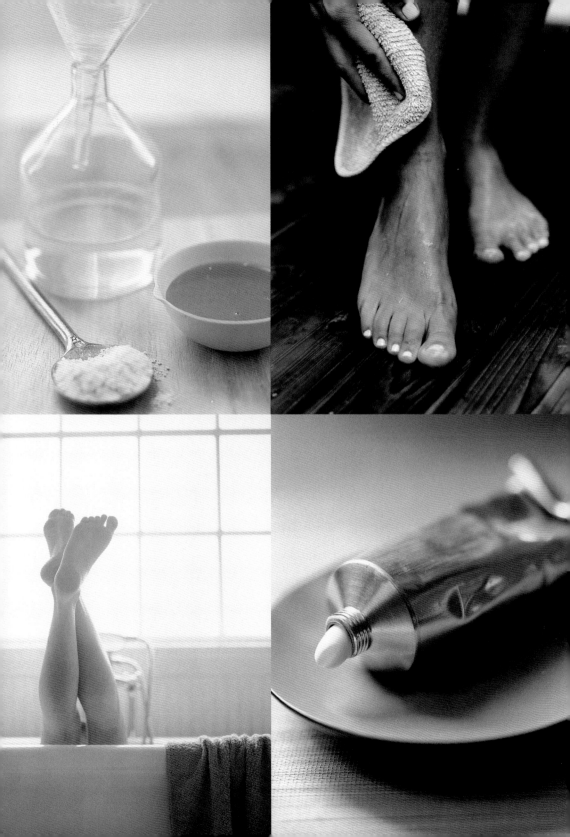

NEUROMA

A neuroma is a pea-shaped mass of nerves that is pinched between two bones of the foot, usually between the third and fourth toes. The pinched nerve becomes thickened and painful. Many patients describe the pain as feeling like they are standing on a cord. Signs of a neuroma include intermittent cramping, burning, and numbness that is aggravated by wearing shoes. Typically, this pain occurs from wearing tight-fitting shoes and can be dramatically reduced by removing the shoe and massaging the painful area.

T R E A T M E N T   Conservative treatment usually includes wearing proper-fitting shoes, orthotics, or arch supports. These conservative therapies may provide complete, partial, or no relief of symptoms. Surgical removal of a neuroma is performed when conservative treatment proves ineffective.

> Wear proper-fitting shoes that have enough room for the toes.

> Modify exercise and physical activities.

SMELLY FEET

Smelly feet, known as *bromhidrosis*, occurs when the foot's perspiration provides optimal growing conditions for bacteria. There is a very high concentration of eccrine glands (sweat-producing glands) in the skin on the sole of the foot. In addition, the temperature inside of a shoe can reach 102° F. Sweat is a good media for bacteria to grow in and the bacteria secretes isobaleric acid, which is what causes the odor.

TREATMENT Smelly feet are exacerbated by synthetic shoes that do not breath; vinyl and plastic shoes are notorious for this. However, even well-ventilated shoes need to air out for 24 hours before they are worn again. It is imperative to keep feet dry: Damp feet promote bacteria that secrete odor-causing chemicals. If necessary, change your shoes more frequently, even throughout the course of a day. Socks that breathe are equally important. In addition to providing conditioning and warmth, socks wick moisture away from the surface of the skin. Cotton blends are the best, as cotton absorbs the moisture and certain synthetic materials wick it away.

The most essential remedy for smelly feet is frequent washing and foot powders. You can also buy deodorant soaps and sprays made specifically for the feet. Soak your feet in a mixture of vinegar and water (see page 63). Combine essential oils with your everyday body lotion and apply to your feet after you shower. If all else fails, your doctor can prescribe internal and topical medication to help reduce perspiration on the soles of the feet.

PREVENTION

> Avoid wearing the same pair of shoes within a 24-hour period, giving them plenty of time to effectively air out.

> Wear socks made with cotton-synthetic blend.

> Frequently changing shoes, even throughout the course of a day if necessary, will minimize sweat.

> Apply talcum powder or foot spray to feet and shoes.

> Wear well-ventilated shoes; sandals are best for warmer weather.

> Use a noncaustic fabric deoderizer in your shoes.

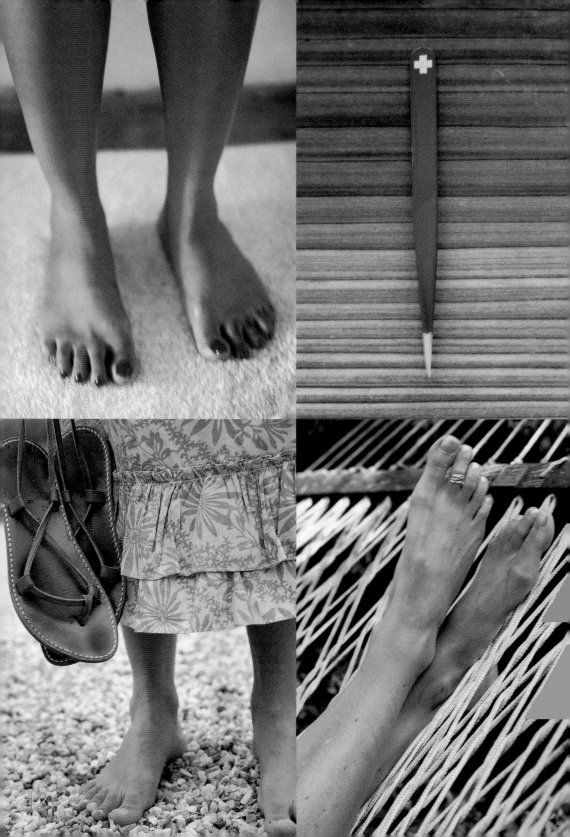

SPLINTERS

Most splinters can safely be removed with household tweezers. The area should be clean, dry, and adequately lit. Do not soak your foot prior to removing the splinter, as this causes the splinter to absorb the water and get larger, making it more difficult to remove. Grasp the end of the splinter with the tweezer and extract along the same line it entered, being careful not to bend or break the splinter. If there is redness around the splinter or pus or other draining fluids, all of which indicate infection, consult a physician immediately and don't try to remove the splinter yourself. After removal, clean the area thoroughly with soap and water and cover with an antibiotic ointment and bandage. Wear soft shoes for a day or two and remember to wear shoes when walking on wooden floors or decks.

SWOLLEN FEET

Feet are known to swell, a condition known as edema, especially in airplanes and warmer temperatures. In the summer, you may notice that your feet begin the day normally, but by day's end they're as puffed up as a peacock. Most often, swelling is a benign condition and is usually due to gravity's effect on fluids. Other factors that cause swelling include high salt intake (salt draws fluid out of the cells and into the spaces between the cells), immobilization, pregnancy, and medication. Swelling can also be the result of a failure in the small valves within the veins of the legs. When healthy, these valves only allow the blood to flow to the heart. If these valves are unhealthy, blood pools in the legs and feet.

Although swollen feet is often a benign condition, it can also be an indication of systemic disease, including kidney dysfunction, diabetes, and thyroid disease, as well as several diseases pertaining to the veins. Consult a doctor if conservative treatments such as elevating your feet above your heart and wearing support socks do not work.

TREATMENT   Keep your feet properly ventilated. As with smelly feet, shoes should be rotated to keep them dry. You want to allow at least 24 hours for a pair of shoes to air out. During a long plane flight you may notice that your feet are prone to swelling, which is due to their immobile, confined position. Walking about the cabin every so often should remedy the problem.

PREVENTION

> Keep feet clean and dry.

> Wear socks or stockings.

> Drink lots of water, especially if you indulge in coffee and alcohol.

> Follow your doctor's recommendations about salt intake.

TOE DISORDERS

The most common toe deformities are hammertoes, mallet toes, curled toes, bone spurs, and overlapping and underlapping toes, all of which may or may not be painful. Corns—a buildup of skin on the affected joint that is often associated with bursitis (inflammation of small pouches, called *bursas,* which lie above the joint between the tendon and skin)—are perhaps the most noticeable and bothersome symptoms. If left untreated, mobility of the toes could be affected and other problems, such as skin ulceration and infection, may develop.

Arthritis, which slowly destroys the joint surface, is another major cause of toe discomfort and deformity. Toe deformities can be aggravated by restrictive or poor-fitting shoes worn for a prolonged period of time.

BONE SPURS

A bone spur is an overgrowth of bone that may occur alone or along with a hammertoe. Commonly found on the sides of the toes and on the heel,

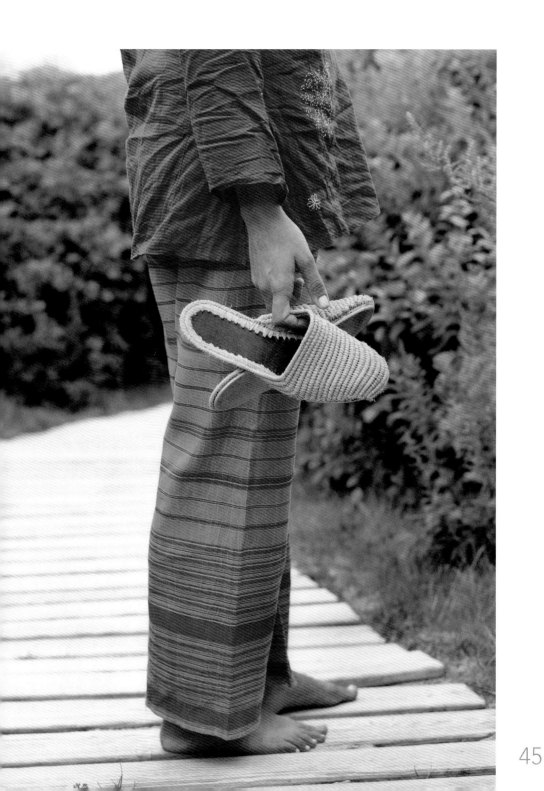

they cause painful lesions called soft corns. Calluses are another major symptom. Left untreated, a bone spur may eventually be accompanied by bursitis or a small skin ulceration. (See Heel Spurs, page 36.)

MALLET TOES

Mallet toes and claw toes are similar in appearance to hammertoes, but affect different joints in the toe. The joint at the end of the toe buckles in a mallet toe, while a claw toe involves abnormal positions of all three joints of the toe.

OVERLAPPING AND UNDERLAPPING TOES

Toes can overlap or underlap each other because of ill-fitting shoes, an untreated bunion, a genetic imbalance of the tendons, or a congenital condition of the bones within the toes. Pain, inflammation, and small corns may result. This interferes with the normal function of the foot and, if left untreated, may lead to enlargement of bone spurs.

TREATMENT Less advanced conditions featuring only minor discomfort may be treated without surgery. This usually involves:

> Trimming or padding corns and calluses

> Wearing supportive orthotics in shoes. This helps relieve pressure and allows the toes and major joints of the foot to function more appropriately by preventing pronation.

> Splints or small straps to realign the toe

> Wearing shoes with a wider toe box

In certain cases, anti-inflammatory medications may be injected to relieve pain and inflammation. Medications have proven to be successful in relieving the discomfort associated with bursitis. While conservative treatments provide temporary relief of symptoms, they may not correct the deformity and surgery might be required.

TOENAIL DISORDERS

Nail problems can be caused by improper trimming, minor injuries, or just being clumsy. Some nail disorders, such as ingrown nails, can also be congenital. In their protective role, nails bear the brunt of daily activities. All or a portion of the nail plate can be damaged when the feet are injured or abused.

CUTICLE INFLAMMATION

Inflamed cuticles, also know as *paronychia*, occur from excessive pressure on the skin. This can result from a too-rigorous pedicure or constantly picking at your cuticles. Infection can easily occur if not treated.

TREATMENT   Inflamed cuticles can be self-treated by soaking feet in a warm bath and applying moisturizing creams. If the inflammation remains after a few days of this treatment, your doctor may prescribe antibiotics. If badly infected, a podiatric surgeon will need to drain the affected area.

PREVENTION

> Cut your nails straight across.
> Don't pick at your cuticles.

FUNGAL INFECTIONS

Most fungi are harmless until they penetrate the skin. A fungus can invade through minor cuts or after an injury that causes the nail to separate from the nail bed.

When a fungus has found its way into the nail bed, the nail may thicken and become yellow or brownish. As the fungus grows, foul-smelling, moist debris that is dry, white, and has a cheeselike consistency is produced. Pressure from a thickened nail or the buildup of debris may cause pain.

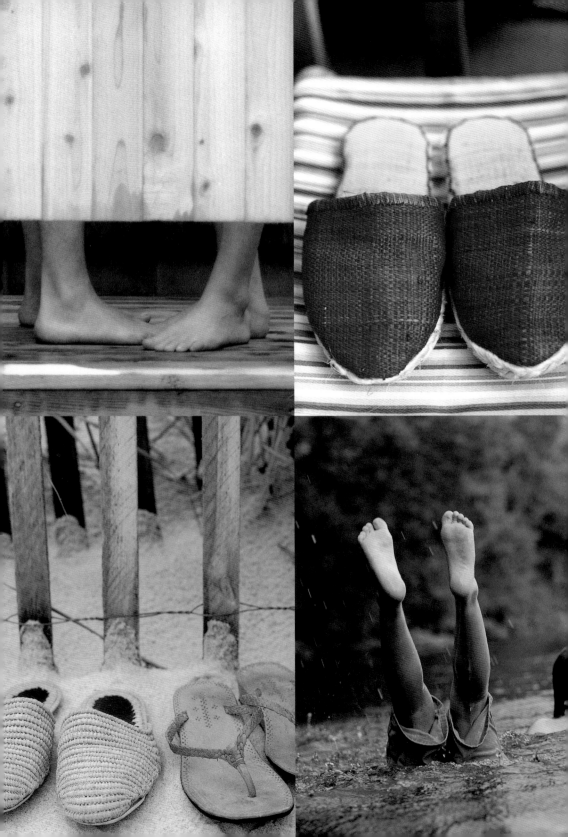

TREATMENT   Naturally, it is best to treat the fungus in its earliest stages of infection. Treat athlete's foot (see page 20) as soon as possible and look out for discoloration along the tip of the nail. Left untreated, the accumulation of debris under the nail plate can lead to an ingrown nail or to a more serious bacterial infection that can spread beyond the foot.

To reduce the pain of a thickened, infected nail, a surgeon files the nail plate down with a surgical burr. Filing will not, however, prevent the infection from spreading.

Oral medication can be prescribed to eradicate the fungus. This medication can have side effects and is not for anyone with liver problems. Your podiatric surgeon should monitor the results of oral prescriptions.

HEMATOMA (BLOOD BENEATH THE NAIL)

A common result of an active lifestyle is a hematoma, or blood beneath the toenail. Hematomas are especially common among people who jog or play tennis, when the toes repeatedly rub against the inside of a shoe. However, a hematoma might also indicate a fractured bone, especially after an injury. Any time you see blood beneath the toenail, see a podiatric surgeon for proper diagnosis and treatment.

TREATMENT   Because hematomas are a result of excessive rubbing against the shoe, it is important to wear thin but cushioned socks and comfortable shoes. If the hematoma is treated within the first few hours of forming, the podiatric surgeon will create a tiny hole in the nail plate. This releases the blood and relieves the pain and is itself a painless procedure. Following this simple drainage, the toe should be soaked in warm salt water and treated with topical antibiotics.

If left untreated and several days have passed and the blood clot becomes painful, the nail plate may require removal so that the nail bed can be cleaned. Some podiatric surgeons prefer to remove the nail plate whenever blood forms beneath it because the blood can promote bacterial growth and lead to infection. A couple of weeks after surgery, the body will generate a hardened skin covering to protect the sensitive nail bed. When this covering has developed, normal activities can be resumed. Nail plates that have been removed will grow again within three to six months.

PREVENTION

> Wear shoes with a large toe box.

> Wear socks that cushion the toe but do not add bulk.

> Treat hematomas promptly by draining the blood clot. Often it can save the nail.

RIDGED NAILS

Ridged nails are usually the result of internal traumas such as high fevers or stress; or external stresses such as too-tight toe boxes on shoes and repetitive physical stress from running or exercise. Similar to the bark rings of a tree trunk, the nails reflect stresses of the body and mind but these ridges may not show up until several months after the trauma has occurred. The ridges will grow out as the nail grows.

TREATMENT The only treatment is to *gently* file the nail flatter, being aware that it will thin the nail plate. You can also use topical nail-ridge fillers sold over the counter.

YELLOW NAILS

When your nails turn a dusky honey color, it could be an indication of a variety of stresses. A fungal infection, pressure caused by ill-fitting shoes, or strenuous exercise are all potential culprits. To determine the cause, your podiatrist needs to analyze a sample from the nail. If the discoloration came about around the time you took up running or began wearing a new pair of pointy shoes, it shouldn't take too long to figure out the source of the trauma.

TREATMENT   If your doctor diagnoses a fungal infection, he or she will prescribe either a topical cream or oral medication. Since it takes at least three to six months for a toenail to grow out, regardless of what ails it, be prepared to wait a while before it is back to normal.

PREVENTION

> Treat a fungal infection at its first onset so it does not spread to the nails.

WARTS

Most often seen on the bottom of the foot, warts usually appear as soft spots that are red, gray, brown, or black. They are typically gray or brown with a center that appears as one or more pinpoints of black. Warts are caused by viral infections that typically invade the skin through small cuts and abrasions.

Though warts are highly treatable, they can nevertheless be quite painful. Because they most commonly appear on the plantar surface, or sole of the foot, they are known as plantar warts. Most warts are harmless and are often mistaken for corns—layers of dead skin that build up to protect an area that is being continuously irritated.

Plantar warts tend to be hard, flat, and rough on the surface with well-defined boundaries. They are generally fleshier when on the top of the feet or the toes. The plantar wart is often contracted by walking barefoot on dirty surfaces where the virus lurks. The virus propagates in warm, moist environments, which is why many people associate warts with communal bathing facilities such as gym locker rooms. It is therefore important to keep the feet clean and dry.

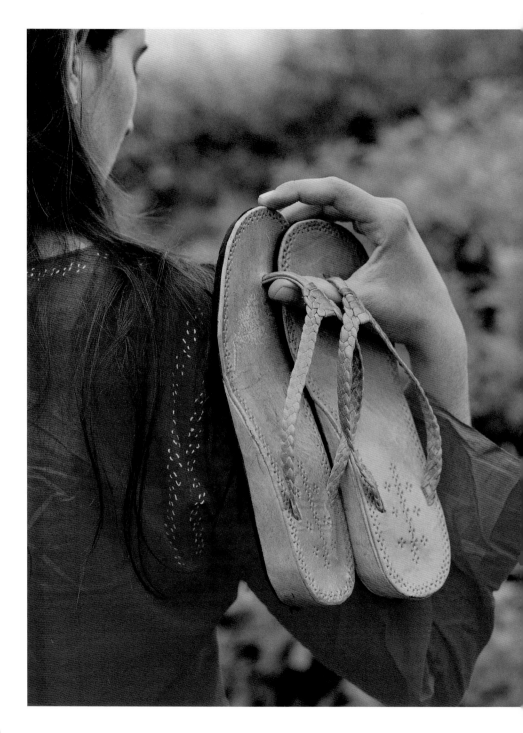

Warts can grow to an inch or more in circumference and spread into clusters of several warts. As with any other infectious lesion, avoid direct contact with other people as well with as other parts of your own body. If the wart bleeds, be especially careful not to allow the infected blood to touch any other areas of the body.

Warts can last for varying lengths of time, but the average is about 18 months. Occasionally, they spontaneously disappear after a short time. Just as frequently, they can recur in the same location or elsewhere.

When plantar warts develop on the weight-bearing areas of the feet—the ball of the foot or heel, for example—they can be the source of very sharp, burning pain. Pain occurs when weight is brought to bear directly on the wart, although pressure on the side of a wart can also be painful.

TREATMENT   Before attempting a remedy, it is sensible to consult a specialist about any suspicious growth on the feet. Your podiatrist may wish to prescribe and supervise your use of a wart-removal preparation. Another option is to remove the wart by a simple surgical procedure.

One common way to remove a wart is to freeze it off with liquid nitrogen, or another process known as cryocautery. Often a second application, some days after the first, is required, and occasionally additional treatments are necessary. Another removal process is electrocautery, which destroys the wart by burning it with an electric needle.

PREVENTION

> Avoid walking barefoot on unclean surfaces. For example, wear flip-flops in public bathing facilities.

> Keep feet clean and dry and change your shoes daily.

> Avoid direct contact with warts.

> Do not ignore skin growths or changes in your skin.

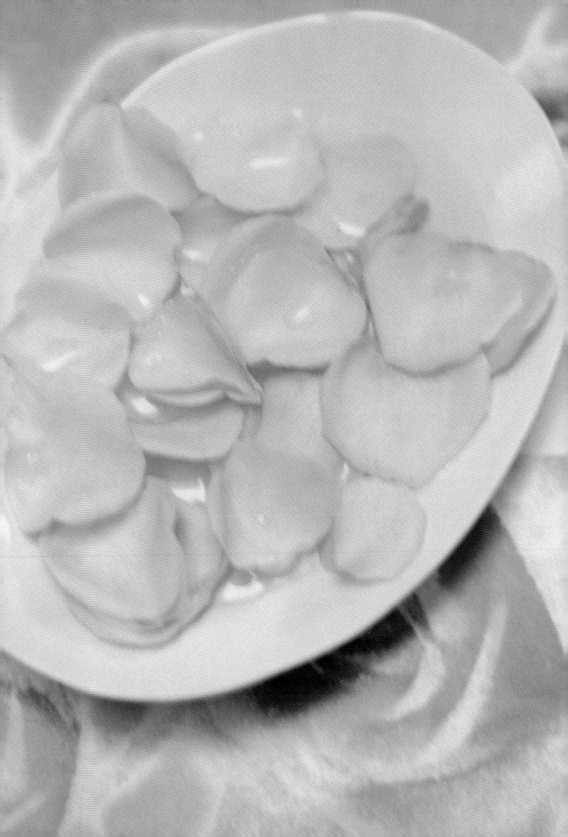

step 3
pampering

HOMEOPATHIC BEAUTY

Now that you know about the harsh conditions that plague our feet, here is the welcome antidote. Consider Step 3 as the holiday after a tough workweek. It's easy to give yourself an effective foot treatment with a relaxing foot bath or pedicure, and it's a sure way to make yourself feel like royalty.

Pampering your feet not only makes them look and feel better, it helps keep them healthy. Along with maintenance, it's the best preventive measure that you can take, allowing you to leave those foot problems in the past. Foot care can be easy and even fun. Papaya, peppermint, honey—the ingredients read like a vegan's grocery list. Going the all-natural, homeopathic route means fewer trips to the pharmacy, and the treatments are as effective as anything store-bought or spa-administered.

FOOT BATHS

To begin, bundle yourself in a fluffy bathrobe, slide in a relaxing CD, and light some candles. You've just created your very own spa at home and have saved yourself a bundle of cash.

A foot bath can be messy, so we recommend that you stay in the bathroom to make cleanup a little easier. Foot basins can be conveniently placed on the floor of your tub and the rim makes a handy seat (with a cushy bath towel under your derrière).

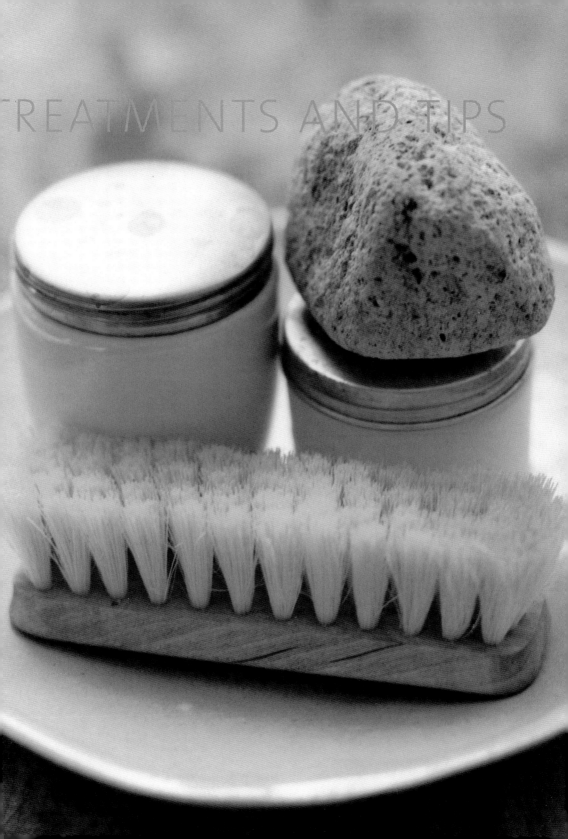

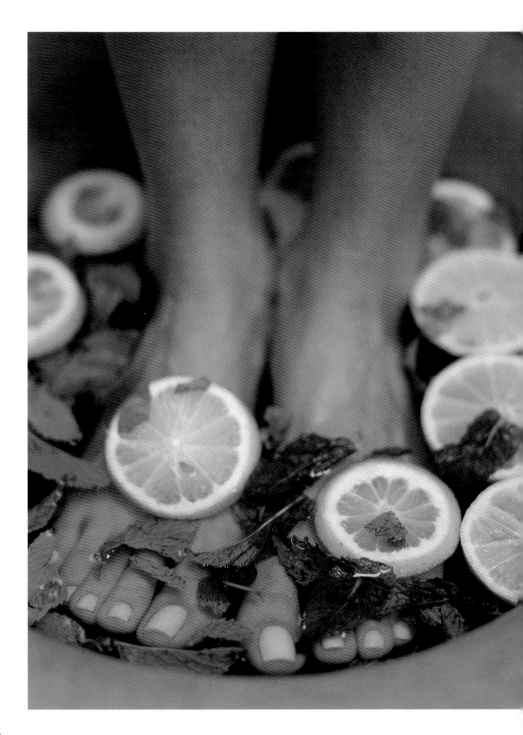

Suggested Reading: While soaking your feet, try reading the *Kama Sutra*. When your soak is done and your pampered feet are ready for display, you may be so adventurous as to try some of those foot techniques with your partner.

NATURAL FOOT-BATH INGREDIENTS

Following is a list of ingredients commonly used in foot baths along with their natural properties.

Almond oil ❯ Soothing and moisturizing properties

Aloe vera oil ❯ Antibacterial; soothing and healing properties

Apple-cider vinegar ❯ Antibacterial; antifungal and anti-inflammatory properties

Arnica cream ❯ Reduces trauma and bruising; anti-inflammatory properties

Blue chamomile ❯ Deodorizing properties

Calendula oil ❯ Great for sensitive, easily irritated skin; soothes rough, flaking, and dry skin

Camphor oil ❯ Freshening, toning, and anti-inflammatory properties

Chamomile ❯ Antibacterial and antifungal properties; soothing and moisturizing effects

Cocoa butter ❯ Moisturizing and soothing properties

Coconut oil ❯ Emollient, moisturizing properties

Dead Sea or Epsom salts ❯ Detoxifying properties; improves circulation

Eucalyptus oil ❯ Disinfecting and skin-purifying properties; cools and soothes

Ginger > Stimulating, revitalizing, and rejuvenating qualities

Grapefruit-seed extract > Antibacterial and antifungal properties

Green tea > Antimicrobial skin refresher and anti-inflammatory properties

Honey > Retains moisture

Horse chestnut > Anti-inflammatory properties and stimulates circulation

Jojoba oil > Emollient, moisturizing properties

Lemon juice > Mild astringent, anti-inflammatory properties

Magnolia buds > Deodorizing properties and creates an energizing sensation

Milk > Moisturizing and soothing properties

Olive oil > Hardens cuticles, softens skin

Papaya > Dissolves dead surface skin cells, rejuvenates skin

Peppermint oil > Stimulating, anti-inflammatory, and antiseptic properties

Primrose oil > Alleviates skin problems associated with itching and irritation

Rose petals > Reduces odor and softens skin

Shea butter > Stimulates circulation; emollient, moisturizing properties

Soy protein > Helps even out skin pigmentation

Tea with tannic acid > Infection-fighting properties

Tea tree oil > Bacteria-fighting properties

Witch hazel > Soothing skin astringent

Caution: If you are a diabetic or suffer from circulatory problems, consult your foot specialist before using any of these treatments. Diabetics are predisposed to infection

ATHLETE'S FOOT

Give your feet a soak that has as much impact as a Sampras tennis serve. The therapeutic properties of this soak, along with doctor-prescribed topical creams, is the best way to beat athlete's foot. You'll need:

Foot basin

2 bags chamomile tea

2 bags green tea

2 drops grapefruit-seed extract

1/2 cup apple-cider vinegar

1/4 cup fresh lemon juice

Tea tree oil

Prescription cream

ESTIMATED TIME: 30 MINUTES

Bring a pot of water to a simmering boil and pour into foot basin. Add leaves from chamomile and green teas, grapefruit-seed extract, vinegar, and lemon juice.

Allow water to cool to a comfortable temperature and soak feet for approximately 20 minutes. Remove feet from bath and pat dry. Swab a cotton ball with tea tree oil and dab onto affected areas. Let dry.

Apply any creams recommended by your doctor.

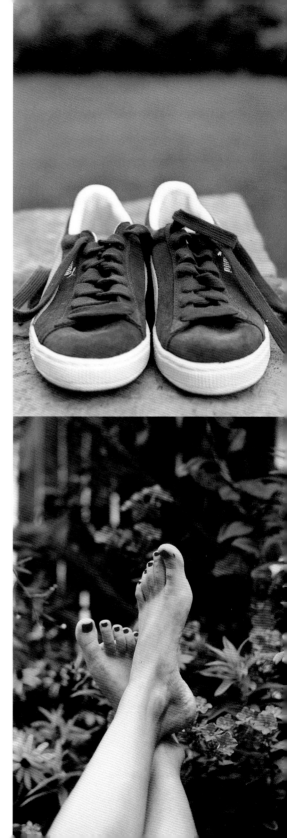

CHAPPED FEET

If your feet are as chapped as lips after a night of kissing a bearded beau, this soak is the perfect salve. Dry, chafed feet should be attended to daily by scrubbing with a pumice stone. Moisturize and wear special socks over creamed feet before you go to bed. Add a weekly foot soak for extra softening. You'll need:

> Foot basin
>
> 1 cup dry oatmeal
>
> 1 cup freshly mashed papaya
>
> 1 teaspoon honey
>
> 2 tablespoons Epsom salt
>
> 1/2 cup olive oil
>
> Half gallon whole milk
>
> 2 drops almond oil
>
> 2 drops tea tree oil
>
> Pumice stone
>
> Emollient cream (such as shea or cocoa butter)
>
> 2 warm towels
>
> ESTIMATED TIME: 30 MINUTES

Before taking the plunge, file toenails into a square shape. Gather your post-treatment tools, such as pedicure accessories, nail polish, and two fluffy towels. Regine Berthelot, senior aesthetician of Frédéric Fekkai Beauté de Provence, suggests heating a towel in the microwave for approximately 20 seconds right before you wrap your feet in them for a little extra luxury.

TO MAKE THE EXFOLIATING SCRUB In a large mixing bowl, combine ½ cup oats, ½ cup papaya, honey, 1 tablespoon Epsom salt, and roughly ¼ cup olive oil. Set aside for use after the soak.

TO MAKE THE SOAK Heat a half gallon whole milk, a little water, and the rest of the olive oil to a comfortable temperature. Pour the mixture into the foot basin and add ½ cup of oatmeal, ½ cup of papaya, 1 tablespoon Epsom salt, and a few drops of almond and tea tree oils.

Soak your feet in the milk bath for approximately 20 minutes. Then massage your ankles and feet with the oatmeal scrub, rubbing vigorously over chapped areas. Return your feet to basin to soak for another 5 minutes. Using a cotton swab, apply tea tree oil on distressed areas and then moisturize your feet with shea or cocoa butter. Wrap feet in warm towels for 5 minutes so that the moisturizer is fully absorbed.

HEEL PAIN

If you have a love affair with all things sexy, sultry, and stiletto, you may be approaching a heated breakup. But before giving your favorite shoes some time off, this soak will chill you out a bit. You'll need:

Foot basin

2 drops peppermint oil

18 ice cubes

Arnica cream

Warm towels

Pillow

ESTIMATED TIME: 45 MINUTES

Fill the foot basin with enough ice water to cover the heel. Add a few drops of peppermint oil. Soak your heels, adding ice cubes (2 or 3 at a time) every 5 or 6 minutes over a 30-minute period.

Apply arnica cream, wrap feet in warm towels, and prop them up on a pillow. Use your condition as a medical reason to watch some bad television. Soak regularly, especially after any physical activity.

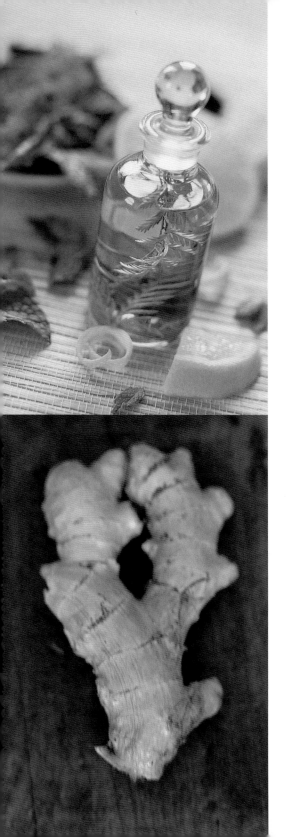

SMELLY FEET

It may be hard to admit that your feet smell bad, but do yourself—and those around you—a favor and take that first step. It is a common condition and, like excessive perspiration or sweaty palms, a normal indication of stress and nerves. Wearing shoes made out of synthetic material (as opposed to leather) or not wearing socks can also lead to smelly feet. Here's what you'll need to have those stinkers coming up roses:

Foot basin

1 bag chamomile tea

1/2 cup apple-cider vinegar

1 tablespoon sea salt

Fresh ginger, peeled and sliced

Magnolia buds

2 drops eucalyptus oil

2 drops peppermint oil

Rose petals

Sponge (preferably natural)

Peppermint soap

Witch hazel

Peppermint foot cream

ESTIMATED TIME: 30 MINUTES

Add chamomile, vinegar, salt, ginger, magnolia buds, oils, and rose petals to basin of warm water. Sponge feet with soap and soak for approximately 20 minutes. Dry feet and then spritz with witch hazel. Finish with peppermint cream.

SORE FEET

After being sore toward someone, it's only considerate to make amends with a thoughtful gift. When you're hard on your feet, that gift should come in the form of a soothing foot bath. You'll need:

Foot basin	1 to 2 drops primrose oil
1/4 cup olive oil	Witch hazel
2 tablespoons Epsom salt	Arnica cream
4 drops eucalyptus oil	Shea butter
2 teaspoons fresh ginger, peeled and sliced	ESTIMATED TIME: 30 MINUTES
1 to 2 drops peppermint oil	

TO MAKE THE TREATMENT In a mixing bowl, combine olive oil, Epsom salt, 2 drops of eucalyptus oil, and ginger. Set aside.

TO MAKE THE SOAK Fill a foot basin with warm water and add 2 drops of eucalyptus oil and the peppermint and primrose oils. Soak your feet for 15 to 20 minutes.

Massage olive-oil mixture into your feet, rubbing into distressed areas. Dip feet back into the basin to remove excess oils and salt.

Dry feet off, spritz with witch hazel, and then apply arnica cream. Once the arnica cream has fully penetrated, moisturize with shea butter.

SWEATY FEET

Don't sweat it: Alternately plunging your feet into warm and then cold water cures excessive perspiration and revives your entire body. You'll need:

2 foot basins

4 bags black tea or tea with tannic acid

3 tablespoons sea salt

1/4 cup apple-cider vinegar

Juice of 2 lemons

Lemon slices (optional)

Handful fresh peppermint leaves

8–10 ice cubes

Peppermint foot spray

Talcum powder

ESTIMATED TIME: 25 MINUTES

Empty the contents of the tea bags into a foot basin and fill with boiling water, salt, and vinegar. Fill a separate basin with cold water, lemon juice, peppermint leaves, and ice. Allow the hot water to cool slightly, then soak your feet in the warm water for approximately 10 minutes and in the cold water for 3 to 5 minutes. Dry feet and apply foot spray and talcum powder.

SWOLLEN FEET

When your feet swell to the-head-of-a-diva proportion, a warm foot bath with green tea, rose petals, and a fistful of stones is the best treatment. It decreases puffiness and creates an overall feeling of well-being. Quite simply, it just rocks! You'll need:

Foot basin

Handful of smooth pebbles or stones
(available at most gardening shops and florists)

2 drops eucalyptus oil

2 drops camphor oil

2 bags green tea

Handful rose petals

1 cup olive oil

Pumice stone

Witch hazel

Arnica cream

Aloe vera cream

ESTIMATED TIME: 50 MINUTES

Place pebbles at the bottom of the foot basin. Coat the stones with eucalyptus and camphor oils. Tear open the tea bags and mix contents with 2 cups boiling water, then pour into basin. Add rose petals and olive oil. Let cool about 5 minutes. Soak feet for 10 to 15 minutes.

Pat feet dry, then buff dead skin with a pumice stone. Trim evenly across with a toenail clipper and file evenly. Massage the bottoms of your feet using the pebbles. If they have cooled, warm them up in the microwave for approximately 20 seconds. Dab your feet with a cotton ball swabbed in witch hazel. Dry your feet with a towel and then rub them with arnica cream until it's fully absorbed. Apply another coat of aloe vera cream, wrap with warm towels, and relax for about 5 minutes.

FOOT-AID KIT
What to keep on hand for perfect feet:

> Cotton balls

> Cuticle pusher

> Cuticle remover
(without phermaldhyde)

> Emery board

> Foot basin

> Foot lotion

> Microwave
(for heating stones and towels)

> Nail brush

> Petroleum jelly

> Pumice stone

> Smooth stones

> Toenail clippers

> Towels

PROFESSIONAL PEDICURES

Just as after a visit to a salon should not be wasted on a night watching reruns, a new pair of open-toe shoes should never be worn without a proper pedicure. Having a professional pedicure is that indulgent perk that actually seems quite practical considering you have someone rub, clean, and polish your feet. However, it is important to select a reputable salon that properly sterilizes their instruments as a precaution against the foot conditions discussed in Step 2.

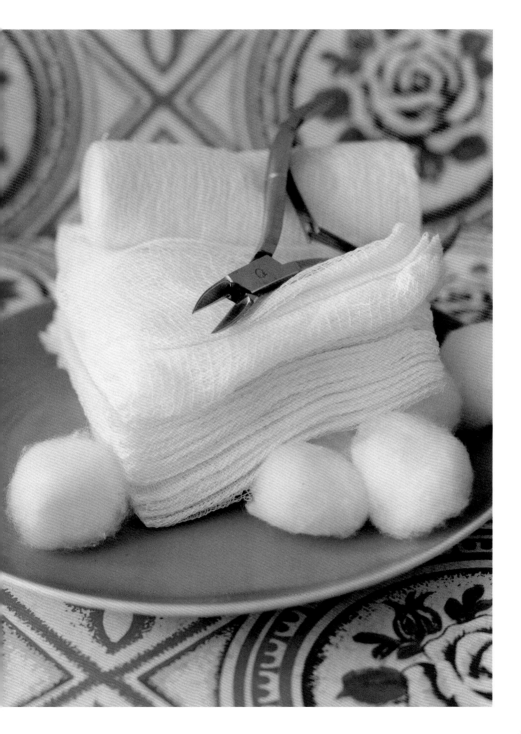

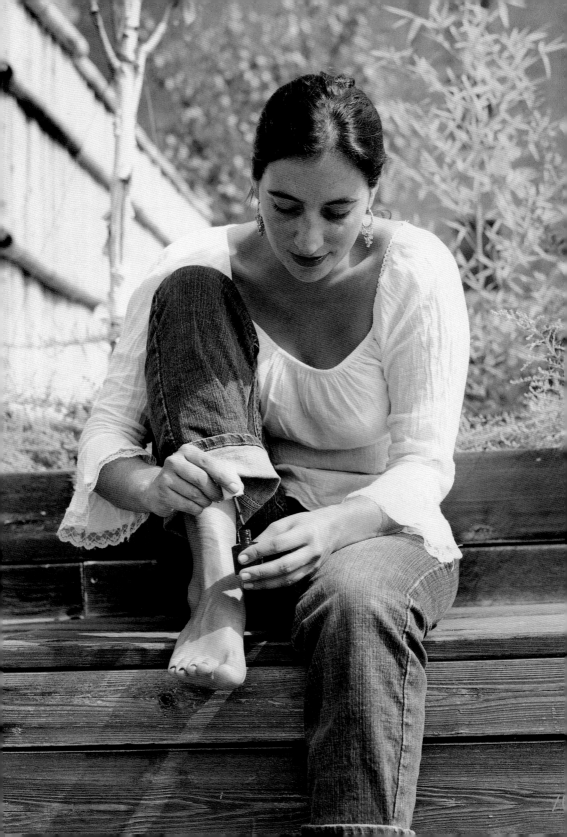

Marcia Kilgore of Bliss Spa in New York City says that it takes a certain level of financial backing to operate a clean, pleasant, and well-run facility. "It would be difficult to operate a great spa at a 'discount' level. I'm not saying that every place has to be fancy, but if the management isn't constantly on top of the details, the quality of any spa can quickly take a dive," she says. Good spas offer everything from polite, well-trained technicians to the highest quality products. "If you don't have these basics," says Kilgore, "a spa experience is not relaxing on any level."

The typical nail bar may not be worth the money you think you're saving. Kilgore urges bargain shoppers to notice how clean the tables are and whether the tools are sterilized.

PROFESSIONAL PEDICURE PRECAUTIONS

> Bring your own instruments and disinfectant for the foot basin.

> Remain loyal to a salon where you've observed high standards of cleanliness.

> Do not allow a pedicurist to use a razor or blade to cut your corns or calluses.

> Get to your appointment early to see how thoroughly the basins are cleaned. After they are washed with detergent, basins should be sprayed with a bactericidal, fungicidal, and virucidal disinfectant.

Pedicures should last between four and six weeks. To maintain that shiny, new-pedicure look, allow fresh polish to dry for at least 45 minutes, pumice regularly, and buy your own polish for touch-ups.

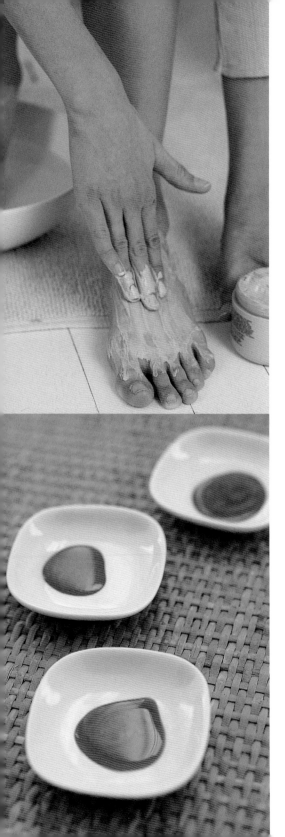

AT-HOME PEDICURES

What you'll need:

> Cotton balls

> Cotton swabs

> Cuticle pusher

> Emery board

> Emollient cream

> Exfoliating cream

> Foot lotion

> Nail polish

> Nail polish, base coat

> Nail polish, clear top coat

> Nail polish remover
(without phermaldhyde)

> Petroleum jelly

> Plastic wrap

> Pumice stone

> Toenail clippers

> Toe separators

> Towels, warm

ESTIMATED TIME: **60** MINUTES
Why not plan a pedicure around watching your favorite television show?

TEN-STEP PEDICURE

After old polish is completely removed, cuticles pushed, and feet are thoroughly cleaned (see page 74), follow these ten steps for perfect toes.

1   Slough off dead skin by rubbing feet with a pumice stone. (Do not cut calluses or dry skin—the more you trim, the more likely the skin will grow back thicker.)

2   Clip toenails straight and then use an emery board to smooth any rough edges.

3   Massage your feet with an emollient cream or use an exfoliating lotion if the skin is rough or dry.

4   Wrap feet in plastic wrap and then a hot towel for about 15 minutes. The heat will help the cream penetrate the skin.

5   Separate your toes with either cotton balls (one between each toe) or toe separators made especially for pedicures.

6   Apply a base coat and allow enough time to dry (approximately 10 to 15 minutes between each coat of polish).

7   Apply polish, attending to any stray marks with a cotton swab dipped in polish remover, then wait till dry. Because there is a greater amount of pigment, the darker the polish color, the longer it takes to dry. In fact, dark polish can take up to 24 hours to dry completely. Also, creamy polishes tend to chip more than those with metallic flecks.

8   Add a second coat to strengthen color.

9   Finish with a top coat of clear polish. The equation is about four coats applied at 15 minutes each.

10 Once nails are fully dried, about 60 minutes, apply foot lotion and massage.

CUTICLE CARE

Incorporate moisturizing your cuticles into your daily ritual. For healthier, more vibrantly colored toenails, soak your feet in warm water for 20 minutes to half an hour with a little salt to aid the circulation. Soaking the feet also softens the cuticles, making them easier to work with during a pedicure. Bathe feet in warm sudsy water with your favorite bath soaps or choose a custom foot bath with warm water (see pages 56 to 67). With a cuticle pusher, gently push the cuticle back wherever it touches the nail plate, using tiny circular movements. Hold the stick at an angle so that you do this gradually and carefully, without going inside the cuticle. This also allows the nails to breathe.

MOISTURIZED NAILS

It is advisable to give your toenails a break from constant polishing. Nails absorb some of the pigment from nail polish and can turn yellowish. For beautiful, shiny, natural nails, put away your purse and invest a little of your time. For nails that are already soft, rub them with petroleum jelly and then buff with a soft cloth. To moisturize nails as dry as a weathered seashell, soak your feet in warm olive oil for 20 minutes.

NAIL POLISH REMOVER

New York City dermatologist Dr. Debra Jaliman recommends using a nail polish remover without phermaldhyde, which causes an allergic reaction for some people and tends to have a drying effect on the nails and cuticles. Avoiding frequent polish changes helps keep the nails moist and healthy. The more often you change your nail polish, the drier your nails will become.

FOOT MASSAGE

Begin by saturating your hands with moisturizer or massage oil. Bringing your sole up to face you, place the fingers of both hands on the top of the foot, thumbs on the heel, and crisscross your thumbs, then work upward toward your toes.

Press your thumbs back on the heel and pulse.

With your other hand on the toes, weave fingers through the toes to the pinky toe.

Work on the ball of the foot with the thumb, move to the middle of the foot, then the lower part.

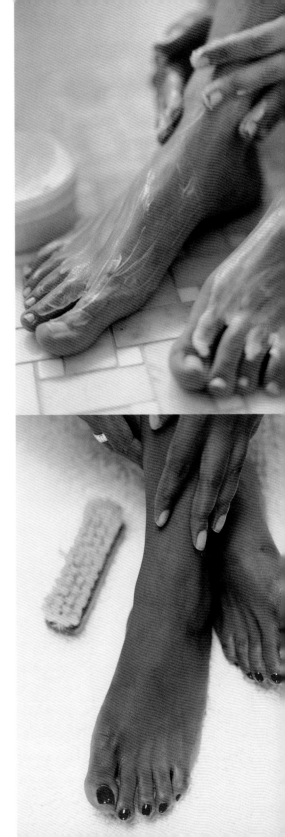

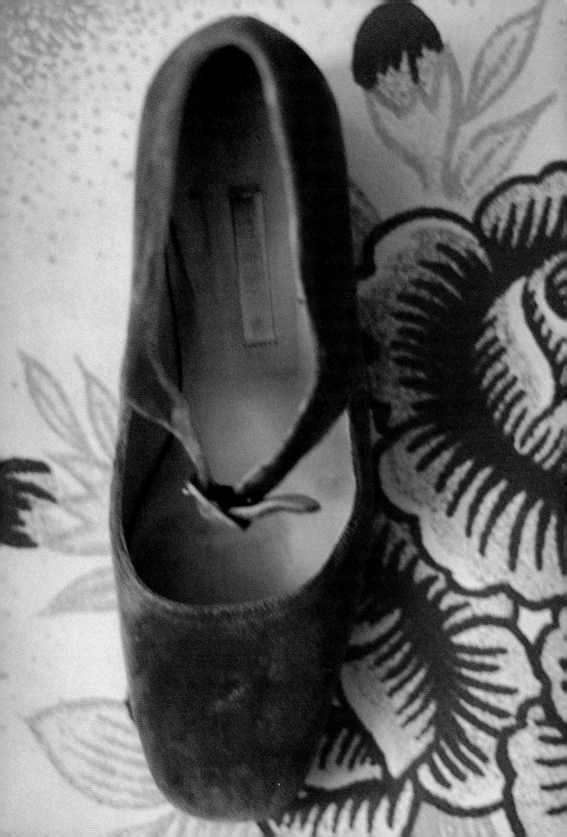

step 4
shoes

CHOOSING THE RIGHT

Crammed closets and depleted bank accounts are just a few of the consequences that may result from a woman's devotion to shoes. While it's easy to become a slave to our shoes, don't allow your feet to suffer the consequences. The majority of foot problems result from wearing poor-fitting shoes, which are made for an ideal foot that doesn't exist in reality. The best way to be a slave to your shoes without feeling like one is to ensure a proper fit by knowing your foot's shape and choosing well-made shoes.

DETERMINING THE RIGHT FIT

Three out of four Americans experience foot problems in their lifetime, but only a small percentage of the population is born with these problems. It is neglect and often poor-fitting shoes that bring on problems. Only Barbie can fit into a pointy stiletto without the pain and discomfort that inevitably accompanies wearing them. For the rest of us, wearing a pointy pump forces the foot into an unnatural position, cramming the little toes into a tiny space and forcing the entire weight of the body onto the ball of the foot.

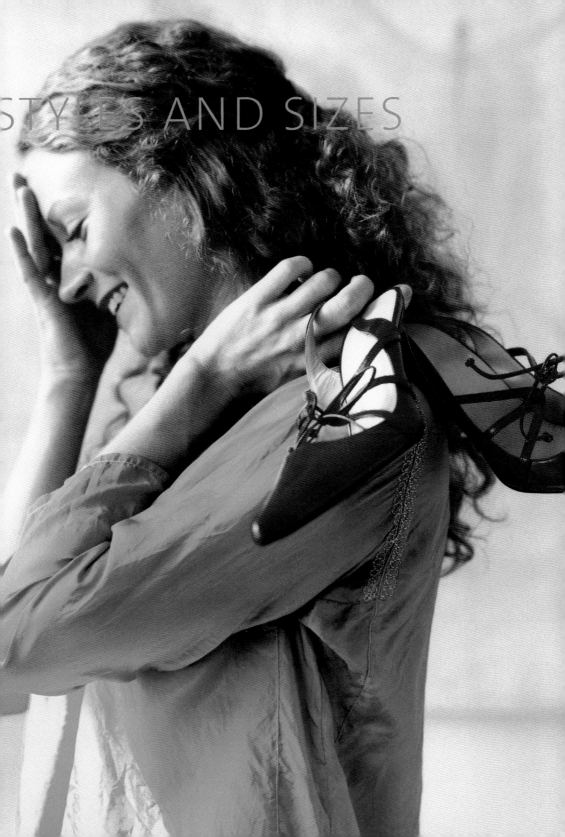

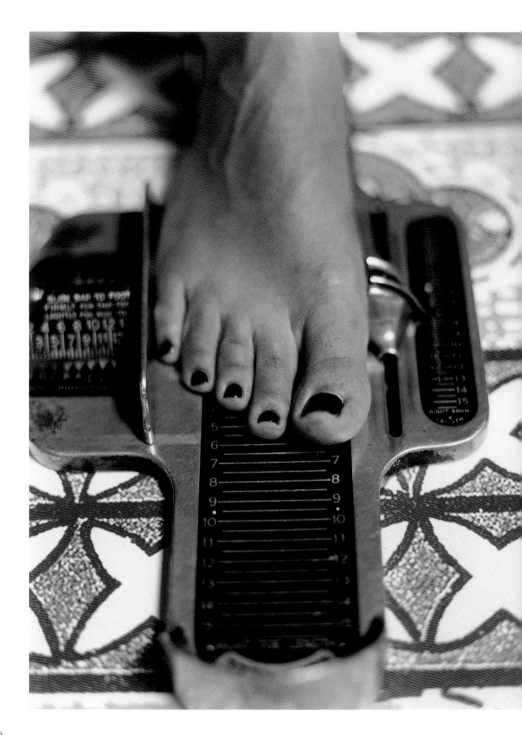

The National Shoe Retailers Association, the American Orthopedic Foot and Ankle Society, and the Pedorthic Footwear Association have jointly published the following "Ten Points of Proper Shoe Fit":

1. Sizes vary among shoe brands and styles. Don't select shoes by the size marked inside the shoe. Judge the shoe by how it fits on your foot.

2. Select a shoe that conforms as nearly as possible to the shape of your foot.

3. Have your feet measured regularly. The size of your feet changes as you grow older.

4. Have both feet measured. Most people have one foot larger than the other. Fit to the larger foot.

5. Fit at the end of the day when your feet are largest.

6. Stand during the fitting process and check that there is adequate space ($3/8$ to $1/2$ inch) for your longest toe at the tip of each shoe.

7. Make sure the ball of your foot fits comfortably in the widest part of the shoe.

8. Don't purchase shoes that feel too tight, expecting them to stretch to fit.

9. Your heel should fit comfortably in the shoe with a minimum amount of slippage.

10. Walk in the shoes to make sure they fit and feel right.

Again, for all those fashion victims out there: Don't sell yourself on a shoe by saying it will stretch out after a few wearings. If those shoes aren't comfortable in the store, it's just not meant to be.

THE ANATOMY OF THE SHOE

1 > INLET

2 > TONGUE

3 > EYELET

4 > LACE STAY

5 > VAMP

6 > SOLE

7 > TOE BOX

8 > WELT

9 > SHANK

10 > QUARTER

11 > HEEL COUNTER

12 > INSOLE

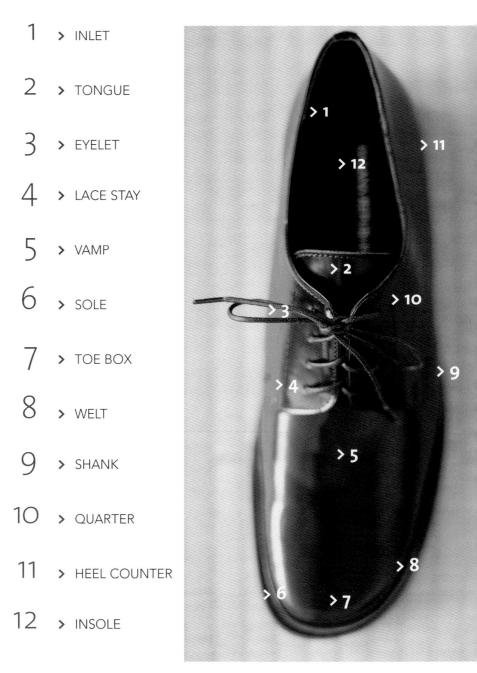

CHOOSING THE RIGHT SHOE FOR YOUR FOOT TYPE

A good shoe fits the foot comfortably, with the right amount of room in the toe box and across the vamp. The shoes should be strong and supportive. If your feet are different sizes, buy shoes to fit the larger one. In Step 1, we showed how to determine your foot type by silhouetting wet feet in sand or on a piece of cardboard (see page 16). You will need to determine whether you have a flat foot or high-arched foot in order to choose the right shoe for your type.

FLAT FOOT

People with flat feet should wear shoes with rigid heel counters. The heel counter will hold the heel in a more vertical position.

HIGH-ARCHED FOOT

A high-arched foot has to handle shock absorption and flexibility. The sole should be flexible and made of materials that are well suited to absorb shock—such as crepe rubber, foam, and EVA (a lightweight rubber of various thicknesses and hardnesses).

CHOOSING THE RIGHT SHOES FOR THE RIGHT ACTIVITY

THE OFFICE

If you are the type who thinks Gucci stilettos look great in the office, be prepared to suffer great pain on your commute to work, not to mention plenty of foot problems after hours. In addition, as anyone hailing a cab during rush hour can attest, heels don't hold up to potholes and city grates. We realize that practical alternatives for the commute, such as the stockings-and-sneakers look (catalogued in recent fashion history along with leg warmers and shoulder pads), just don't cut it anymore, so we recommend a low-heel sandal, loafer, or driving moccasin, which works fine without looking too *Working Girl*.

Once at work, it's sensible to kick off those stilettos beneath your desk, allowing feet to breathe.

BACKLESS SHOES

Backless shoes—which include mules, slides, slingbacks, and thongs— require the feet to sustain the friction needed to keep the shoe on. As a result, the feet are prone to chafing and dry heels. And don't forget to apply sunscreen.

FLATS

While flats may not have the sexy sleekness of a stiletto, they do have the comfort edge, which in turn can bolster confidence and promote the kind of lasting beauty that comes from within.

By placing weight more evenly over the entire foot and allowing more space in the toe area, flat shoes prevent bunions and hammertoes from becoming irritated. However, be sure to avoid those flimsy ballet-slipper shoes that not only skimp on height but also on support, which can result in conditions such as *plantar faciitis* and inflammation of the arch.

EVENING

When going for glam, high heels and stilettos work best for traipsing the red carpet.

High heels do something for a woman's physique that leaves a flat simply *flat*. The heel accentuates the leg's length, which no amount of leg lifts

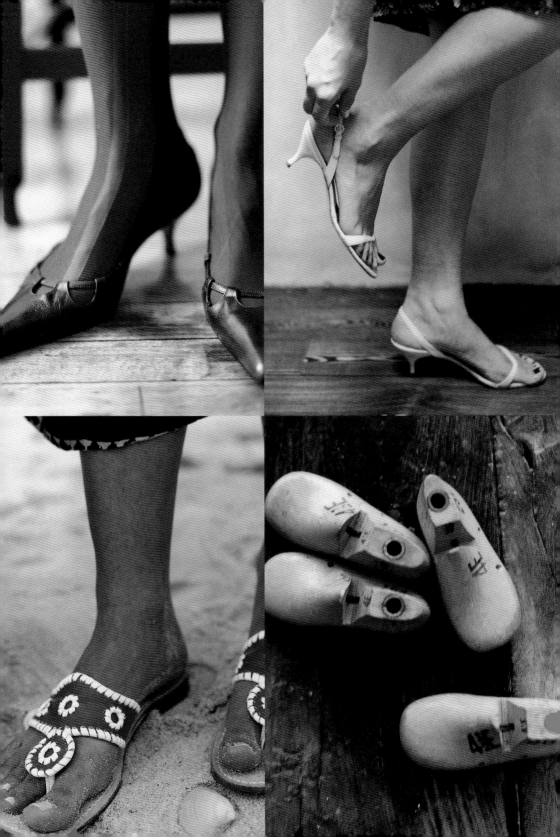

could achieve. They pitch your weight forward, pushing the chest forward and the rear end outward to create an overall J. Lo-on-Grammy-night curvaceous effect. Unfortunately, they also put excessive and unnatural pressure on the foot.

Heels not only put the calves under strain but also put more pressure on the balls of your feet. For those prone to developing calluses and inflammation on the balls of their feet, high heels will only aggravate the condition. Walking in heels also increases your chances of ankle sprains and tripping. Luckily, not every night is worthy of an Oscar performance, so save stilettos for special occasions.

ATHLETIC SHOES

COURT SHOES

Any sport that demands quick movements, side-to-side lateral movements, and some bounce will demand a court shoe. Tennis, basketball, volleyball, squash, and other racquet sports all require court shoes, which are flexible while stabilizing your feet.

Court shoes are usually designed with flatter soles, a firm heel counter, and a padded toe box that helps prevent the injuries that commonly plague tennis players.

RUNNING

While the selection in running shoes may rival the choices in the dress shoe department, you are not going for style here. The demands put on your feet during a run are three times greater than walking. As the heel strikes the ground, its impact is typically two and a half times your body weight, an impact that also puts stress on your ankles, knees, and lower back. Running shoes are specifically designed to redistribute and absorb shock to lessen the stress felt by these joints.

The main types of running shoes incorporate motion control, stabilizers, and cushioning. It is recommended that you change running shoes every 350 to 500 miles or every six months to maintain proper shock absorption and help prevent injury.

The best materials for a sneaker are leather, suede, and canvas, as they are the most durable and breathable materials. Synthetic materials don't allow the foot to breathe, and contribute to skin diseases and foot odor.

SKI BOOTS

Ski boots are the most important piece of ski equipment, therefore it's wise to purchase from a reputable sporting goods store or ski boot shop with an experienced fitter. (No browsing on Ebay for deals on this one.)

A ski boot should feel firm, supportive, and tighter than your normal footwear. When you try on a ski boot, fasten the boot so tightly that you cannot wiggle your toes but not so tight as to cause them to become numb. Unfasten your buckles between ski runs to rest your feet. You will notice most professional skiers do this before getting on the lift.

Less is more when it comes to socks, so don't double up. Socks made with polypropylene or cotton-synthetic blends keep feet warmer, wick moisture away from the skin more effectively, and further decrease the likelihood of blisters than either wool or cotton. Carry extra pairs to change into if your socks become too damp.

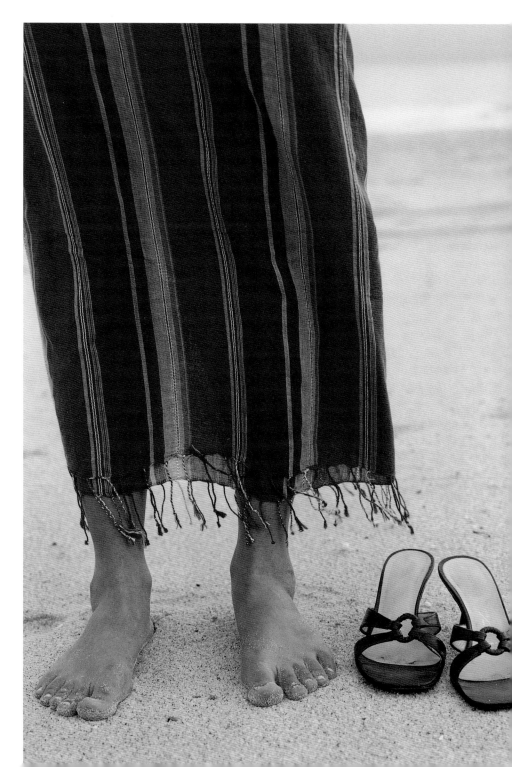

BAREFEET

Going barefoot allows your feet to breathe. There's also less friction, you are less likely to develop calluses, and it's a great excuse to show off your pedicure. The risks are that you are more susceptible to developing plantar warts and athlete's foot, as well as cuts, scrapes, and any other mishaps that can be prevented by wearing shoes. After walking barefoot, wash feet thoroughly with warm soap and water. So, as signs direct, there is a right and wrong time to go barefoot.

ORTHOTICS

Orthotics are special shoe inserts that help properly align the body. People with flat feet use them to aid in the transfer of the gait's flexible phase into the rigid phase by controlling the subtalar joint (see page 16). Orthotics keep the foot in a neutral position, the most efficient position to support and transfer weight. They also reduce shock, relieve areas of excessive pressure, and cushion and stabilize the foot.

Those who need orthotics include people with chronic diseases, notably arthritis and diabetes, and those with bunions, tendonitis, heel pain, and high and fallen arches. An orthotic also acts as a temporary stabilizer after surgery or a sports injury and is used as a preventive measure when performing athletic activities. Your podiatrist will be able to determine whether or not you are a candidate for an orthotic.

Orthotics can be purchased over the counter in various molds; otherwise your podiatrist will prescribe a custom-made orthotic.

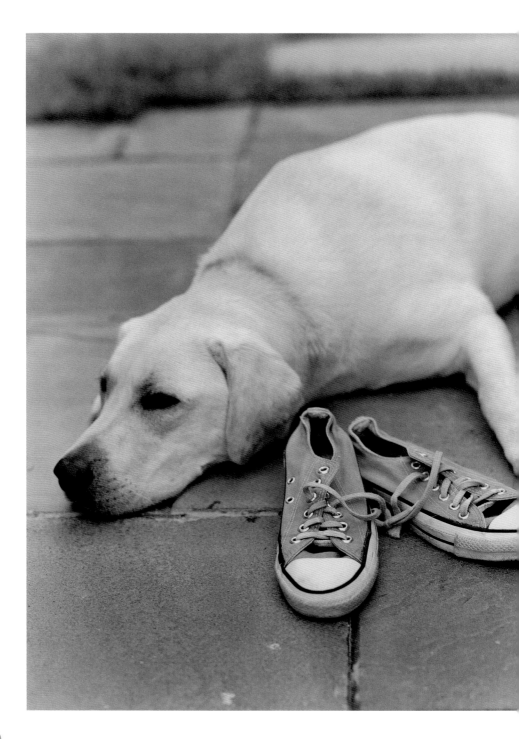

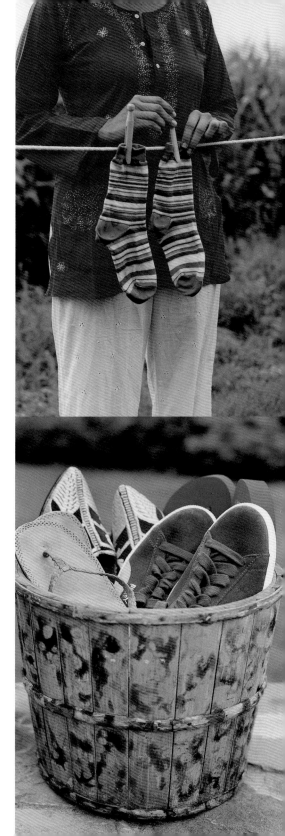

SOCKS

Socks decrease the friction between your feet and your shoes, protecting them from calluses, blisters, and sores. The skin of your feet has to be dry to breathe, and socks can help absorb that moisture or wick it away.

Change socks frequently if you perspire heavily. Cotton blends, which keep feet dry and protected, are best.

TIME TO TOSS

A shoe's expiration date is not signaled only by its questionable scent. A typical gait lands on the outside of the heels, which wears out this side of the shoe. When the heel is obviously worn down along the outside, it's time to either replace the heel or get a new pair. If the heel counter collapses or is no longer stiff, the shoe should be replaced, since this is usually not reparable.

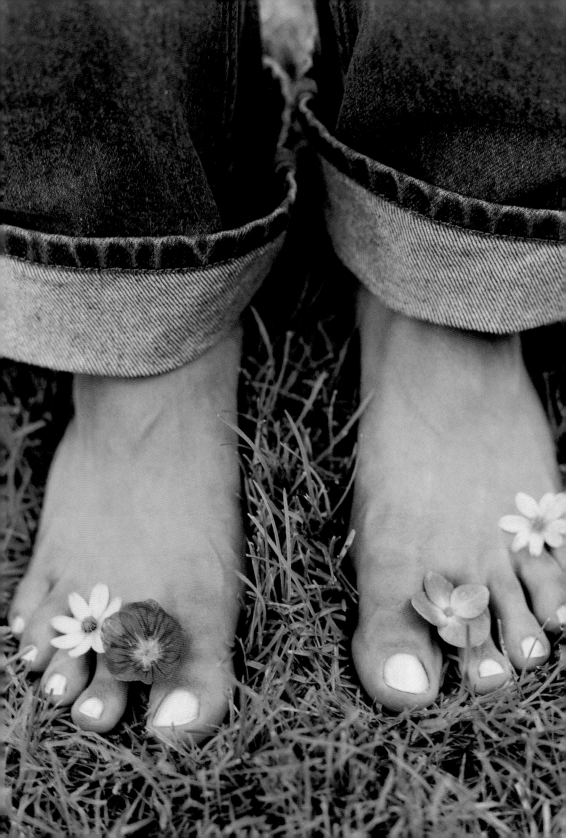

step 5
everyday

TEN FOOT STEPS

1 Check your feet for lumps, bumps, blemishes, grazes, and cuts, and treat these imperfections at their first onset.

2 Wash your feet at least once a day, and always after exercise.

3 Keep your feet warm and dry.

4 Trim your nails straight across.

5 Exfoliate your feet with a pumice stone.

6 Apply a moisturizer to your feet at night and then put on socks so that the moisturizer fully penetrates your skin.

7 Don't covet shoes you can't wear. Instead, go shopping for ones you can.

8 Insure that your shoes fit properly—there should be approximately the width of your thumb between the end of the longest toes and the end of your shoe.

9 Alternate shoes so you will have dry, clean shoes each morning.

10 Stretch (and not just after sports).

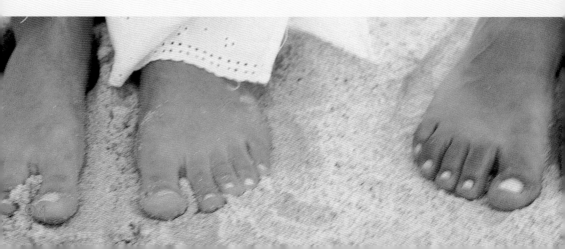

A FOOT TALE

It was during gym class—back when physical abilities were tested in sessions of tumbles, sit-ups, and pull-ups. What was once a welcome break from multiplication tables is now a hyped gym class replete with $1,500 annual fees and an eye-patched instructor named Itzak with a following of other one-name models and musicians.

Separate lines of girls and boys formed outside the locker rooms, merged together, and congregated on cushioned mats that had the stench of musty basement air. Barefoot, stealing awkward glances of classmates' feet before the next round of exercises—if this scenario were to be psychoanalyzed a therapist would have a lot to work with. I was, am, plagued with two webbed toes and the information was about to go public.

Up until that gym class this was never an issue of insecurity. I was programmed not to perceive these attached little toes as an abnormality but rather an extraordinary sign of how special I was. When I first stumbled onto my toes' skewed composition, my mother had an instant, probably rehearsed, answer that webbed toes were a sign of royalty.

When I was confronted by an impertinent Eric Simmons on my two glued toes, my mark-of-a-princess tale was met with the kind of hysterics only second-graders can muster. Defiant, I maintained a proud defense for my toes that never let on to the despondence that genuinely overcame me concerning this sticky little matter.

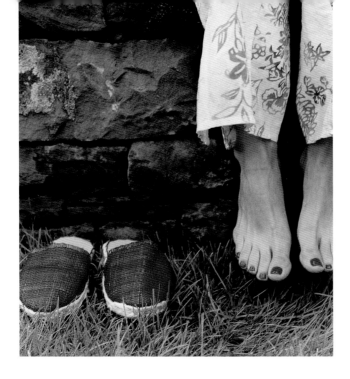

I survived the ridicule, was comforted by my royal stature, yet the issue arose again one Christmas when I was unable to fit into the latest trend, which came in the form of groovy rainbow socks with their own toe slots, like fingered gloves for the feet. After much pulling and failed insertions that took the stocking stuffer concept a bit too literally, my mother again had just the right solution and did some simple tailoring. A few snips and stitches later I began my own fashion trend—the four-toed sock—that could not be easily duplicated.

Now back in present-day 21st century with some years to rationalize these childhood traumas, I am still comforted by mother's original story regarding the illustrious origin of my particular deviation. Every little girl wants to grow up to be a princess and, if less than perfect feet is my assurance to this position and considering that Prince Charles is not an option, so be it.

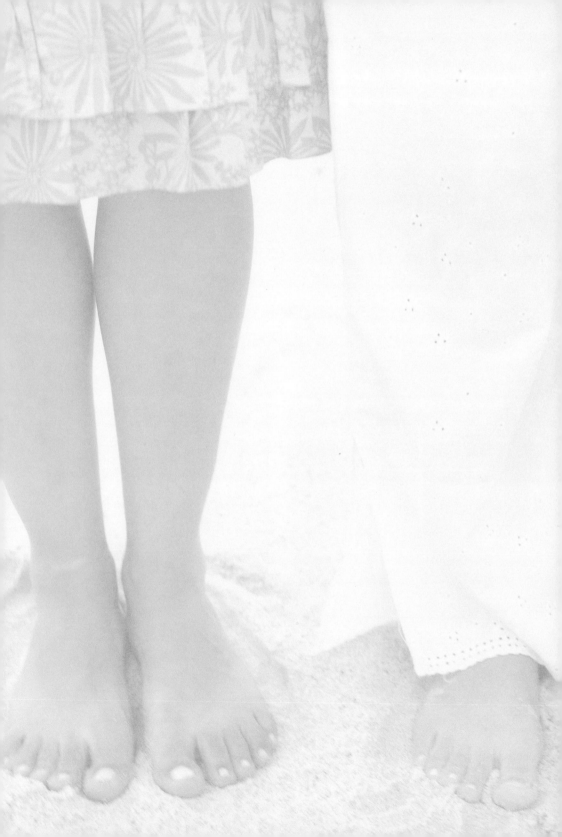

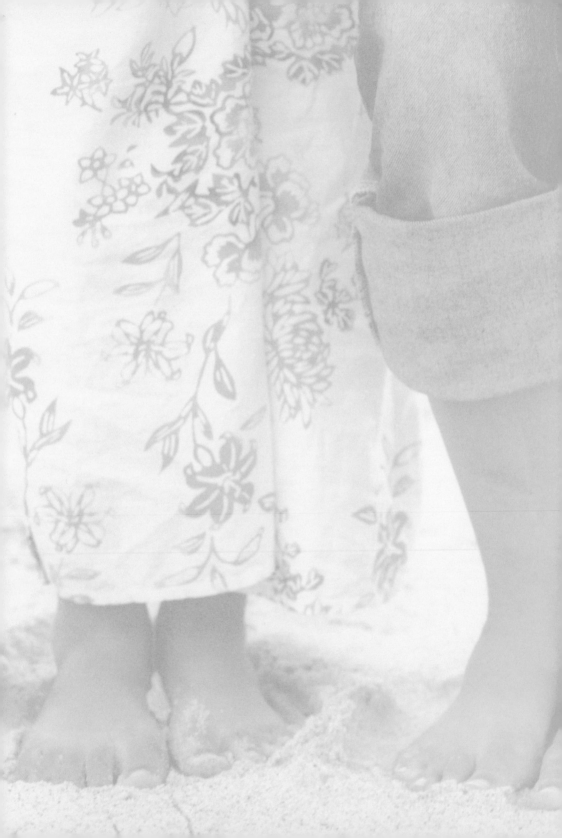